OPENING NIGHT

OPENING NIGHT

The Complete Guide to Producing Christian Drama

LAURA HARRIS SMITH

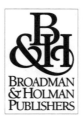

BROADMAN
& HOLMAN
PUBLISHERS

Nashville, Tennessee

© Copyright 1993 • Broadman & Holman Publishers
All rights reserved
4275-29
ISBN: 0-8054-7529-X
Dewey Decimal Classification: 808.2
Subject Heading: Drama—Technique
Library of Congress Catalog Card Number: 92-44629
Printed in the United States of America

Library of Congress Cataloging-in-Publication Data
Smith, Laura Harris, 1965-
  Opening night : the complete guide to producing Christian drama / by
Laura Harris Smith.
    p.   cm.
  ISBN 0-8054-7529-X
  1. Dinner theater—United States.   2. Church entertainments.
I. Title.
PN2270.D56S6   1993
792'.022—dc20   92-44629
                                                                    CIP

For
Granny Rooks

Special Thanks

The people mentioned here have given of themselves in a very personal way to see to the publication of and the inspiration for this book. How I wish they could all have their names on the front cover! Primarily, I am indebted to my friends at Broadman. Thanks also to the supportive staff at the **First Baptist Church of Donelson, Tennessee,** and my visionary pastor and friend, **Dr. Roy Fisher.**

And from my heart, I thank all the **original cast and crew members** of *The Inȼentive* and *The Healing*. Wherever you all are now, I pray God's blessing on you for what you added to His kingdom and to my life. To **Trish Morrison,** I say thank you for answering my many questions: sometimes twice! Thanks to the **Friday Night Adult Bible Study** and the **Monday Night Youth Bible Study** groups for caring enough to pray weekly for the publication of this book. Naturally, I'm indebted to **my parents and my brother and sister** for their attendance at every public performance, and their undying attention during every private performance they were ever forced to endure! Thanks for clapping.

Finally, I turn my heart toward my own precious family. To my husband **Chris,** I thank you for sharing my burden to reach a dying world through God's dramatic Word in the only way I know how. I thank you also for being such a great daddy to our four children, **Jessica, Julian, Jhason,** and newborn baby **Jeorgi Anna,** who wrote this book with me and waited to make her debut into this world until only days after its completion. I love each of you individually and what we are together.

> "And I thank Christ Jesus our Lord who has enabled me, for that he counted me faithful, putting me into this ministry" (1 Tim. 1:12)

PREFACE

Two thousand five hundred years ago, Drama was born. Did you know Drama was that old? If you answered that you thought Drama had been around even longer, since the beginning of time, perhaps you are right. After all, Drama imitates life, so as long as there has been life, there's been Drama! Still, everything dates back to an origin or a date of creation, and Drama is no exception. But more on that in a minute!

Dinner theatre is another genre that has been around for a long while but is suddenly bursting forth onto the scene in churches everywhere. Whether you have this book because you are in a church that desires to minister through dinner theatre, or a school or other organization wanting to raise money producing plays, the contents here were written with your every question and need in mind. Enclosed are two plays to get you started.

For the church, Drama is an incredible ministry tool that is barely being tapped into. The churches that use it, use it a lot. Those who don't, think it's too difficult to organize any form of drama. For you pioneers who will read this book and really put it to use, encourage others to do the same and teach them how if you must. There are a scattered few who believe that drama has no real place in the church, perhaps due to its origin. The story began in ancient Greece over 2500 years ago, when the Greeks worshiped a god called Dionysius (the god of fertility, etc.) and their worship included singing dithyrambs, or chants, to him.

One day, a fellow named Thespis decided these chants were completely unorganized, so he lined one group up ''here'' and one group up ''there'' and cued them when to chant. Pretty soon, unknown to them, they were organized actors being directed by their leader, Thespis, and the first ''thespians'' were born. Of course, there isn't a lot we can do today to change the origin of a wonderful art form born out of a pagan ritual 500 years before Christ. The truth is, drama couldn't have been born any other way. Besides, God can use anyone, or anything, regardless of its origin!

Pagan rituals aside, the church cannot deny that the Scriptures cry out with dramatic action. Why, Jesus Himself was the most dramatic man to walk this earth... His entrance into this world, the telling of His parables, the giving of His Father's miracles, and, of course, the sacrifice of His very life. As Christ left this world and early churches were being formed to educate the first Christians, Drama was banned within the church due its pagan origin.

In fact, it would be 800 years before a ninth-century priest would be reading his Bible and feel the conviction to convey God's Word in a more applicable fashion through the use of Drama. The response was more than favorable as many forms of drama thrived within the chruch for the next 500 years. Mystery, miracle, and morality plays hit the scene and set the stage for the next major turn in theatre—the Shakespearean era. Changes in Drama have been steady and rapid in the past few centuries as well. Unfortunately, Drama may well have come full circle back around to the pagan ritual. Today's theatre, films included, are loaded with lewdness and lacking in decency. Regardless of our religious preferences or our family statuses, we must contest this by taking action to balance the "bad stuff" with some new "good stuff." To compete, it must be entertaining and not just educational: thus, the inspiration for this book.

Whether you decide to organize your own dinner theatre, or merely produce a play minus the dinner experience, the dramatic needs for your play remain the same. Chapter One, "Drama Q's and A's: Defining Your Format," will help you easily decide if you are able to host a dinner theatre. It is the perfect format for fun *and* fellowship, for laughing *and* learning, and so this book will often refer to dinner theatre due to the recent large demand for information. Dinner theatre is the quickest way to assemble hundreds of people from all age groups, afford them the opportunity to meet new friends, form new relationships, and, hopefully, return to your church. If done well, it will affect your church's growth in a positive way, and so, this book will encourage you to try to organize your own dinner theatre. (Chapters 8 and 9 deal exclusively with Dinner Theatre.)

Still, if you discover that simple play production is more your speed, then read on! This book is a complete guide that has left no stone unturned in helping to prepare you for your first OPENING NIGHT!

With your vision, you can introduce your church to the many faces of Drama. In the same way that music ministries were brought into churches... one church at a time. And perhaps, in a few hundred years, history will record, "and at the end of the twentieth century, churches everywhere reached out to their communities, and they laughed and learned together with the use of a tool called... DRAMA."

Contents

Chapter Breakdowns

1. Drama Q's and A's: Defining Your Format—lists requirements and advantages of dinner theatre to assist reader in deciding on hosting a dinner theatre

2. Choosing a Play—contains a quiz to help reader best define his audience, budget, actors' abilities, and purpose for producing a dinner theatre; suggests where to go to select a quality play

3. Get Ready... Get Set... Write!—an encouraging chapter to the beginning writer including a formula for constructing your first storyline

4. Casting a Play—auditioning processes, plus tips on how to find a place for everyone on either a crew or in the cast

5. The Director's Chair—the ten chief roles and responsibilities of the director

6. Practice Makes Perfect... or Does It?—rehearsals: organization from first read-thru to dress rehearsal; includes sample schedule, techniques

7. Technical Techniques—discusses lighting and sound needs; lists and defines all necessary technical and production crews

8. Creating the Dinner Theatre Mood: A Memorable Experience for All the Senses through music, food, programs, ushers, etc.; ten steps toward a complete dinner-theatre environment

9. The Dinner—Half of Good Dinner Theatre Is Its Dinner!—tips on menu, caterers, small budgets and the covered-dish dinner theatre, kitchen managers, and the actors serving the meal in character

10. Acting—includes an actor quiz on "Discovering Your Character's Objectives"; acting techniques for raising emotions, avoiding tension, and suggestions for character "quiet times" and warm-ups

11. Publicity and Budgeting—areas of budgeting and how to plan for them; pricing and selling tickets for making a profit or breaking even; a total guide to publicity coordination

12. Opening Night—calming your cast through emotional, physical, and spiritual preparations

1

Drama Q's and A's: Defining Your Format

"Theatre in the church?!" ... "You mean, churches are producing comic and dramatic plays beside the typical Christmas and Easter musical?" ... "Could my small church or school group actually produce a full-length play?" ... "What if we don't have access to a stage?" ... "What is Dinner Theatre?"

If these and other questions like them are standing in between you and the production of your first play or dinner theatre play, you are not alone. These very questions spawned the inspiration for creating a production guide that would be more than just another stagecraft manual. A complete guide should address the normal steps of production, such as selecting a play, casting it, directing it, rehearsing it, and then technically enhancing it with lights, sound, etc. However, what about advice on budgeting and publicity? What if a group has searched but has not been successful in locating a quality play? A complete guide would include a couple of plays to get them started, and then encourage and educate them in the steps needed to try their own hand as a playwright. In short, a complete production guide is not complete unless it leaves no stone unturned in preparing a drama group for its first OPENING NIGHT.

Opening Night is the complete guide to producing Christian Drama, or any other form of drama within schools, colleges or other organizations. Today, there are countless forms of drama that can be utilized as teaching tools, ministry aids or just plain fun for your drama group—formats such as clowning, mime, puppetry, improvisation, reader's theatre, seasonal pageants, dramatic creative worship, street theatre, plays (dramas and comedies), and dinner theatre.

This book will address the last two, plays and dinner theatre plays, since the demand for instruction is so great and since the requirements for both are so similar. As you read, keep in mind that *Opening Night* aims to encourage you to organize your own dinner theatre, since so many more people can be reached at one time through its means. "To Dine or Not to Dine" . . . That is the question when deciding on Dinner Theatre! So, how do you know which format is right for you—theatre or dinner theatre? There is only once distinction between good theatre and good dinner theatre and that, of course, is the dinner.

Yet, that one difference introduces an entirely separate area of preparation that you and your group must be mindful of before attempting to give your audiences the best of both. For instance, most of your audience will have paid to see a play at least once, and you can count on the fact that they've all paid to go out to dinner before! Just because many of them have never done both simultaneously is irrelevant, since they will pay good money and show up on opening night, expecting from you the best of both: a satisfying meal *and* a good play.

Within this book is an exhaustive blueprint to the entire dinner theatre experience. You need only to staff the separate committees mentioned and find an adequate space for your play's performance. So, why would anyone opt "not to dine" when deciding on dinner theatre? Why would anyone think twice about hosting such an unforgettable affair?

Simply put, dinner theatre seems like a huge undertaking that only a large group can handle. But the smaller your group, the smaller your drama cast and production will be; and the smaller your production is, the smaller your performance/serving place will need to be. Likewise, with a smaller-scale performance space you will need fewer lights, microphones, and the like. Your production need only be complete, not necessarily extravagant. Also, if you are a small church or organization, and you still desire a large production, then consider consolidating your efforts with members of another small church or group in your area. If none of you can provide the auditorium for a large audience, then find a local, neutral site such as a high-school gym or a nearby park with a covered pavillion. (Make sure you are allowed to rehearse wherever your performance will be held, since rehearsing and performing your play in different locations can be a huge setback to your cast.)

To help you decide whether dinner theatre is for you and your group, let's discuss its requirements and its advantages. The following is a basic list of what you will need to produce a two-act play, such as the ones in this book, within a dinner-theatre environment.

1. *A Director.* A willing person who can organize, motivate, and communicate with people while shaping a play (Possibly you since

you're making the effort to read this book! See Chapter 5, The Director's Chair.)

2. *Willing Bodies.* Enough to cast the play you choose to perform and also others to serve on technical crews—this number can range from 10-40 people, depending on your cast and technical needs.

3. *Performance/Serving Space.* One large enough for (1) a stage or flat area on which to rehearse and perform, and (2) your tables and chairs—A gymnasium can be beautifully transformed into a dinner theatre playhouse, as can a fellowship hall. Any outside area can also host a dinner theatre on the ground as long as you have alternate rain dates scheduled.

4. *A Menu.* Food provided either by a caterer or through covered-dish donations brought in by your audience—Either way, the food is served by the cast, in character! (See Chapter 9, The Dinner)

Those are the four main hurdles to overcome when starting a dinner theatre. There are many other elements, such as plates and utensils, costumes, lights, and sound equipment. But those are minor considerations since disposable plates can be bought, your facility's serviceware can be used, and since a modern-day play (such as *The Inçentive* and *The Healing*) can be performed, eliminating the need to search for and make costumes. Also, depending on how large your performance space is, you may not need such special effects as lights and sound amplification. However, if you do have a large space that demands to be lit and magnified with hidden microphones, then chances are that your church or organization is also large enough to contain within it someone who specializes in this technical field. If you meet the four requirements on the previous list, then congratulations! You can easily start a dinner theatre and host a production as often as your schedule permits. So, let's count the advantages of dinner theatre and see what it can do for you, now that you know what you must do for *it.*

1. Dinner-theatre groups, like any other group of dramatists, bring together young and old alike for a wonderful blend of fellowship and fun during your weeks of rehearsals.

2. You can reach many people at once through a play and its message. If your goal is to bring people into your church or organization, the dinner-theatre environment is a perfect opportunity to make your guests seem right at home.

3. Dinner theatre can be a profit maker! If this is your aim, then charge your customers slightly above what your caterer charges you per plate. For instance, if he charges you $3.50 per person/plate, then set your ticket price at $5 and make $1.50 profit on each ticket. If you predict 100 people will attend your performance(s), then count on profiting $150 to bank or to spend on props, costumes, lights, etc. If 1,000 people will attend your performances, then you'll have $1,500 to save or spend as your group wishes.

Perhaps your group is a non-profit organization and you wish only to break even. In that case, count on a no-frills play and charge each person only what your caterer charges you per plate. Of course, you may wish to avoid using a caterer and have your audience members bring an assigned dish each in exchange for lowering their ticket prices. (Again, see Chapter 9, The Dinner, for more helpful dinner ideas.)

4. Despite all the work, dinner theatre is unbelievable fun! Your time together as a cast will form lasting friendships, and the fruit you all will see from your hours of hard work and talents offered is overwhelmingly fulfilling. Oh, the first production you hold you may have to knock on many doors before finding those "willing bodies." But after just one production you'll be astonished at the people who will call you asking to be a participant instead of a spectator the next time around. Truly, each dinner-theatre production becomes easier and easier.

If, after all your efforts and all suggestions mentioned in this book, you are still unable to produce a dinner theatre at this time, then consider the next two options.

First, don't abandon your desire to produce a play merely because you cannot adequately seat *and* feed a crowd. Only Chapters 8 and 9 of this book deal exclusively with dinner theatre, so if you choose to omit the dining experience for now, that's OK. This manual can still serve you as a theatrical-stagecraft guide, so keep reading! Plus, *The Incentive* and *The Healing*, although written for dinner theatre, easily stand on their own as producible, non-dinner-theatre plays. Although there would seem little need to charge an entry fee for this type of production with no meal, you might consider either a small charge or taking a love-offering to collect the funds needed eventually to fund a full dinner theatre.

Second, if space is not your problem but finding willing bodies is, then contemplate a *dessert* theatre instead. Replace your meal with catered pies and coffees and perform a simple one-act play. (This is a shorter play, lasting about 30-60 minutes, with no intermission.) Dessert theatre productions require fewer cast members and fewer technical crews and will spark the initial interest you need to gain volunteers for an eventual dinner theatre. Again, if you cannot find a caterer, or wish to avoid this route, then ask your cast to bake the pies. Or, request audience pie donations, and have the evening's best pie win a free ticket!

Budgeting can also play a large role in your decision to start a dinner theatre. You may have to convince your church staff or your organization's planning committee that this event won't drain all of their funds. Assure them that you will keep your first production modest and that costs will be minimal. Also, keep in mind that your largest expense will be your caterer and that most caterers send their bills after their services have been rendered, and you have collected your ticket money. Therefore, you really don't have to spend much up front at all, and what you do spend can be reimbursed by your ticket income.

Do all your homework (including finding your caterer, your play, and planning your financial needs) before you make your presentation on starting the dinner theatre. Your pre-organization and step-by-step budgeting will satisfy and calm any fears regarding losing money on the endeavor. There is absolutely no reason why you should lose money, even though your first couple of seasons will be your tightest productions financially.

Persuading your church staff or organization of the benefits of dinner theatre will be much easier. If your goal is to reach the unchurched and convey a message of Christ's love to your audience then summarize your play's theme for your church staff and remind them of what an effective ministering tool drama can be within the church. If the dinner theatre is seen as a possible money maker for you, then convince your group that you can easily control your dinner theatre income by raising or lowering your ticket price to meet your financial needs. Always remember, though, that a fair ticket price ensures a larger audience.

Finally, you should be able to predict by now whether or not you can produce a dinner theatre. If you met the four basic requirements, and you liked the four advantages to dinner theatre, then keep reading! There's no reason why you cannot produce your first dinner theatre production eight to ten weeks from now. After that, you can host more dinner theatre productions at the same rate. This rehearsal schedule, discussed further in Chapter 6, Practice Makes Perfect... Or Does It?, is based on two months of rehearsing, meeting once a week the first month, and then three times a week the second month as your production nears. Allow more or less time and create your own rehearsal rate based on your cast's schedule, of course. Have you read this chapter and opted "not to dine"? Fine for now. Consider the other options mentioned before and start casting a solid play.

Whichever position you find yourself in, continue on to Chapter 2, where we will now explore Choosing a Play.

2

Choosing a Play

Your local cinemas and movie theatres know in advance the movies they will show each week. Your community theatres distribute annual invitations by mail for you to subscribe to and buy seats at their many performances they have planned for the year. Even high schools and colleges plan their productions and select the materials they will perform far in advance.

This, too, is where you must begin, even though choosing your first play may seem like a race in which you can't quite find the starting line. This is understandable in church dinner theatres, since locating quality, full-length Christian dramas can be perplexing. Any drama which contains the Christian message is worthwhile. That goes without saying. Remember, though, that only your mature Christian audience will feel this way. The portion of your audience which is unchurched and classified as non-believers will primarily be seeking entertainment. However, it is your responsibility, if this is the goal for your dinner theatre, to convey underlying themes of God's love in Christ Jesus through the play you select. This means selecting a play in which the characters face everyday struggles and then find realistic resolutions through their hope in God. If the play is a good one, it will be easily related to; that is, it will contain characters your audience can identify with. By following a character's journey with anticipation and sympathy, each audience member will hopefully make the same transformations as the character he or she has identified himself or herself with. This is using drama as a teaching tool and not simply as an entertainment device.

If recognizing and finding good material seem all too easy for you, then you may have an untapped resource which you have not yet discovered. Yourself! There is a huge need in churches for more high-caliber Christian dramas, and you may be exactly the person to contribute to expanding that area by writing your own drama just for your group. This is exactly how *The Incentive* was born. It was the first dinner theatre play performed by the First Baptist Church of Donelson, Tennessee. Notice in it how there are far more women's roles than men's. (This reflects an initial shortage of men when we first began. Thus the play was written with four female lead roles that were easily filled.) Notice also how this play involves a wide variety of ages—from infants to children to youth to young adults and then to the grandmother. (This was intentional since we wanted to help the whole church gain interest in the new concept of dinner theatre.) And on a humorous note regarding *The In¢entive*, pay close attention to the character Cassandra and her exits and entrances throughout the play. Each time she comes and goes she has with her a rather large object, such as a box of sweaters, a tray of food, or some shopping bags. These props were purposeful, you see, because although the actress who played Cassandra was just perfect for the role, she was also six months pregnant, and Cassandra was supposedly unable to have children! Of course, our actress was finally able to shed all of her bulky props in Act II as Cassandra and Owen discovered they were finally expecting a baby! You see, necessity is the mother of invention, and there's no hurdle you can't jump even when you can't find the right play for your group of players. So if you feel you may need to write a tailor-made play to custom fit your unusual drama group, then Chapter 3, Get Ready, Set, Write!, will be helpful to you.

At this point, however, whether you are choosing a play or writing one, let's examine what steps you must take when you are searching for your play or searching for good writing ideas. Begin by taking the following quiz. Answer each of the following questions and give yourself one to three points for each answer, depending on which number answer you choose. (For instance, if on question #1 you chose answer #3, all ages, then give yourself three points. If you chose #2, older audiences, then give yourself a score of two points.)

1. What is the expected age of my audience?
   1. youth of younger audiences
   2. older adults
   3. all ages

2. What is the purpose of my production?
   1. to entertain only
   2. to teach
   3. to entertain, teach, and convey God's truths

3. How much time will my drama team have to rehearse?
   1. minimal time

     2. little to average time
     3. they seem to be flexible

4. What length of play are we searching for?
     1. a very short drama
     2. a one- or two-act play that is relatively short
     3. one or two acts, no matter how long the play is

5. What type of dramatic experience have I had in the past, either as an actor or as a director?
     1. none
     2. some
     3. extensive

Is your score near an average of five? Then look for a simple, short drama with few characters involved. If your score is closer to an average of 10, then search for an average-length play with the content and characters of your choosing.

However, if your score is high and close to fifteen, you and your drama team will have great flexibility. You can be less concerned with a fixed-play length or a limited-rehearsal schedule and concentrate more on the content you desire for your audience. Determine your audience's needs before you select a play. In other words, will they need to be taught or simply entertained? Finding a play that does both provides an unforgettable evening for your audience. Of course, there are other questions to consider, like, do we want a humorous comedy or a serious drama? Will our play be an all-season play, or do we need a seasonal Easter play or Christmas pageant?

By asking yourself "What type of play does my audience need and, what can my drama group handle at this time?" you will narrow the selection process and make it easier on yourself to find the perfect play. Always remember that when ministry is your main dinner-theatre goal, God already has precisely the right play in mind for your group. Your church may be struggling with some inner-relation issues that you are not even aware of—but because God is, He may very well use your dinner theatre format to speak to the church. So, prayerfully asking His help in selecting your play is vital. If you *are* aware of an inner struggle in your church, choose a play that kindly addresses this issue. Remember, though, never browbeat anyone just because they're a part of a captive audience. Comedies are wonderful teaching tools since the audience can identify with the characters and laugh at them, as well as at themselves.

If pure fun and entertainment are the only objectives for your dinner-theatre production, then defining your audience will be a bit more tricky. On the one hand, you are freed up from the instructional responsibilities that a ministering dinner-theatre team has. But on the other hand, you have to predict what type of play will best sustain the interest and entertain the group of people you'll be performing for. For instance, is your audience full of children? Then a Shakespearean tragedy (or even one of his comedies) should not be on your list of plays, no matter how much you want to culturally educate these youngsters. If your younger audience members will have a parent present, then perhaps they can handle a symbolic drama of short length. But remember, part of defining a young audience is remembering that young children have short attention spans. No matter how splendid your performance may be, if it is not brief, you'll be performing to a squirmy, inattentive audience. If your dinner theatre is set on a college campus, then think twice before selecting a play about problems faced by the elderly. After all, youth consider themselves invincible, and they don't think much about their aging years. Also, if college students had to perform such a play, you'd face quite a challenge aging all your actors by 50 years and expecting your audience to suspend their disbelief and buy it!

So you see, selecting a play is no more than a process of questions and answers, mixed with intuitive common sense. Now that you are closer to knowing *what* you want from your play, let's discuss *where* you can go to find it.

Bookstores—Your local bookstore will carry a variety of plays in small-script form. In the front of these small paperback scripts will be a synopsis or preview of the play. This will quickly allow you to view the play's content, as well as its length and the characters within. If you like what you read, then you can order the additional scripts you'll need from a form within that book. Never buy one script and make copies from it. This is an unlawful copyright infringement unless permission to make copies is clearly given somewhere within the script or book.

Libraries—If you are familiar with a particular playwright's work and want to view his various plays, then visit your local library. Again read the play's synopsis and see if its content meets your needs as well as your standards. If the play contains all your needs, such as a certain amount of characters or a desired length, then again look within the book for ordering information. A hardcover library book is unlikely to contain an order form, but it will have publisher's data on the first few pages. Simply contact the author's publisher, and they will gladly help you order scripts, or perhaps charge you a royalty performance fee for performing the play. Again, never make copies directly from the book without expressed permission, since this is an infringement upon the author's rights. Remember, authors make their living when their plays are requested and purchased for performances.

Church Library or Christian Bookstores—These are excellent places to find good, moral plays, but your chances are slim for finding several plays to choose from. What material you do find though, still has the same copyright laws attached to it. Never assume that your church has paid a flat fee for the performance rights to that play. The book may have been purchased for your library, but it's up to you to contact the publisher, or order and pay for additional scripts.

Dramatic Publishing Houses (Publishers)—Here, you can really let your fingers do the walking. Simply call one of the publication companies listed at the end of this book and order one of their catalogs. They cost usually about $2-$3. Once the catalog arrives, you can shop for a play in the comfort of your own home. These catalogs contain hundreds, sometimes thousands, of plays from which you can preview content, length, and characters, and then order the scripts for a fee. Most two-act play scripts are around $5 each. In addition, these publishing companies will charge an average performance fee of $40 for the first performance and $30 for each additional performance. So, if you choose a play with ten characters, you'll need to purchase ten scripts from them and an additional five or so for technical and production personnel, including the director. That's $75 so far. Then, if you plan on two performances, count on an additional $70 in performance fees. So on the average, to perform a two-act play with ten characters is $145. One-act play scripts usually run $2.50-$3.00, and performance fees are generally $20 for the first performance and $15 for each additional show. In short, a one-act play will cost you half as much in performance fees and script costs. Baker's Plays, in Boston, Massachusetts, actually publishes two separate catalogs. One contains secular plays, musicals, and children's dramas, and the other catalog is strictly for religious dramas, of which they are the largest publisher in the world.

After deciding what type of play your drama group and audience need—if you have searched high and low and still cannot find the right play or cannot afford to purchase performance rights to one—then give serious thought to writing one! After all, would it hurt to try? If you fail, you'll still be one step closer to defining your audience, and if you succeed you will have met your group's need as well as some other group that has your unique dilemma (that is, *if* you decide to find distribution for your play through a publisher)! If you write a Christian play and seek publication, you will have helped fill a huge need for church drama troupes like yours all over the country. Are you brave enough to try? Then Chapter 3 is for you!

3

Get Ready...Set...Write!

Up to this point, writing a play for your group has been referred to as some sort of last resort. Actually, it is preferred by many, just like some people prefer to create their own clothes or bake their own bread. Have you ever tasted a fresh, hot loaf of bread, or worn a jacket tailor-made just for you? Both are deliciously inviting and leave you feeling satisfied.

So it will be when your drama troupe reads through a play tailor-made for them. If you really want to include every actor, you can create roles for each of them, keeping in mind that you should never create a character who is unnecessary to your play's plot. Also, don't create characters to match your actors' personalities, or your actors will never get to *act*. Writing a play for your drama troupe's first dinner-theatre production will be easier than writing for any other production you ever present, since we already discussed that your drama group will grow considerably each year as your dinner theatre gains more and more publicity.

Each season, more and more people will audition, and eventually some will not find a place in the cast at all. Instead, they may find a spot in a high-need area such as the production or the technical crew. Whatever the need for your writing, try to find a healthy balance between your group's needs and your reasonable creativity. For example, you may have a wonderful idea about a plot for an all-girls' school, but a drama team of mostly men will not be able to fill those roles! Had you been an actor in one of Shakespeare's plays it wouldn't have mattered. All of his actors were men, and they played all the roles, both male and female. Obviously, his main objective lay in the incredible quality of his work and not in the believability of some sections of his performances. But there's no reason why today you can't accomplish both, so make note of that girls'-school plot for later use and start on another plot better suited to your actors!

Maybe you aren't writing for any particular group of people, but you merely want to write, period! Either way, this chapter will address what quality plays consist of and will help you start on your very first storyline.

Storyline

What is storyline? Perhaps you're more familiar with terms such as plot or theme. However, storyline, plot, and theme are three separate pieces to your uncreated puzzle. Sound confusing? It's not. Storyline might be most simply defined as that first glimmer of an idea you receive for creating a play. Rarely does your "glimmer" appear in a finished fashion, but rather as an intriguing idea on which to build. Stop right now and jot down any "glimmers" you may have. (With these ideas on paper, you can add to them as we progress through the entire chapter.) Early on, you discover an indwelling theme, although some playwrights might begin with a theme and create their storyline around it. Either way, the two combined serve as the perfect cornerstone for your sleeping masterpiece.

To best define storyline, let's not find a one-line formula, but instead let's examine what is needed to build a storyline. Broken down into nine parts, think of storyline as containing all of the following elements:

Setting
Timeless characters
Obstacle(s)
Resolution(s)
Yawless plot
Life-like dialogue
Inherent theme
Natural progressions
Evolution of characters

Setting. Although this is usually the first piece of information given about a story within the first or second page of a script, it is not necessarily the first idea born in a storyline—unless of course, your story is about a certain country, such as the political upheaval in Austria in the late 1930's. Then your setting may be the first thing you decide about your storyline. But there is more to your setting than where your play takes place geographically. What about the central location of the action? Where will that occur? More often than not the main action of the play is set in the surroundings or in the home of your main character(s). This is a sure way to eavesdrop often on the main characters. For instance, in *The Healing* the setting is Brookport, Illinois. The action is set in the home of Emmett Lee Westbrook, a well-known author who is suffering from extreme bitterness and emotional separation from his family after the loss of his wife some twenty years before. Since understanding Emmett's past is the key to unlocking his future, the play is also set in his home of twenty years ago by the use of an alternate, small stage, decorated in the late 1960's fashion and covered with a scrim. This double setting magically transports the audience back in time at any desired moment, and the use of a scrim is a splendid technical surprise. A scrim is a thin piece of woven material that serves as a large drape in front of a stage. When lit from the front, the fabric appears cloudy and opaque. However, when frontal lights are removed and the scene itself is lit from behind the scrim, the scrim becomes transparent, and the audience is allowed to watch the action behind it. This "double setting" also reveals a third section to "setting a play," and that is called *time period*. *The Healing*'s main action takes place in the late 1980's, with flashbacks of the late 1960's. At what time will your play take place? This question is important to your characters' behaviors, the current issues they'll discuss, and the costuming they will require.

Setting (geographical, action and time settings) are vital to your storyline and should be decided upon before you begin the writing process. This adds to your play's realistic qualities, character action, and props needed. For instance, the two plays contained in this book take place within a month of each other in winter, although they're set in different years. So why do characters constantly remove coats and hats upon their entrances and exits in *The Healing* but not in *The In¢entive*? Simply because *The Healing* is set in Illinois and *The In¢entive*, in Georgia. Therefore, geographical factors make the characters in these two plays behave differently. Likewise you should decide on the setting for your play before you ever pen a single word.

Timeless Characters. Certainly your story, its plot, and its theme are very important ingredients in your play. But of equal or even greater importance is deciding who will prepare those ingredients: namely, your characters. Your play must be a perfect marriage between a progressive plot and memorable, timeless characters. One without the other will dilute the delivery of your play's theme, or its central idea.

As promised, we'll discuss plot and theme soon enough, but for now what constitutes a timeless, memorable character? We'll take one adjective at a time, only it should first be stressed that all the characters you create must be a part of propelling your plot. Each character in your play should therefore have his or her own motives, purpose, or identity. This, like real life, makes for an interesting combination of personalities between your on-stage characters during any given scene. How many characters will your storyline need? You do not decide. Your storyline decides for itself, naturally. Within that "glimmer" of an idea you may already be having about your storyline, awaits an exact number of characters needed to carry out the plot. No more. No less. So stop now and let your storyline establish your characters. This comes first. Next, comes defining them.

A timeless character is one who surpasses all limits of time and location. He or she remains easily related to today even if the play takes place 100 years ago. Remember Romeo and Juliet? No? What about Maria and Tony in *West Side Story*? Never saw it? Well then, maybe you caught the same young-love struggles between Danny and Sandy in *Grease*, or between Samson and Delilah in the Book of Judges, or on one of the numerous television programs you may have viewed just this week. The later examples given here are less likely to be copies of an earlier playwright's plot than they are to be mere recaptured, universal, timeless characters who will always find themselves fighting the same battles and telling the same stories. A timeless character is easily related to. True, no single character can relate to everyone, but to keep him vague and neutral in hopes of having him relate to everyone will leave him identifying with no one. This viewer identification process is vital to keeping your audience's interest. What's more, it is the method by which a spectator is entertained by a relatable character and then educated by that character's final transformation or evolution.

Finally, your characters should be memorable. Each should be distinct in both personality and actions. Think of how boring life would be if we were all made from the same mold! So it is with the theatre. Remember the all-girls' school idea? If a good play is to follow that idea, then the conforming all-girls'-school image must be the only thing these girls have in common, shedding it, of course, at key moments to reveal their true selves. Memorable characters should be constant: that is, unwavering and even predictable in their created personalities up until the point of resolution. Your plot should never be predictable, but your characters' basic natures should be for your play to retain its believability. A constant character does experience change during the play's climax and resolution, but keeping his personality steady throughout the play's beginning and middle only adds to a suspenseful ending. Stop now and clearly define the characters you established earlier.

Obstacle(s). No storyline is complete without a conflict. What's more is the significance of introducing it very early within the story. This conflict can be defined as your story's question, or *what you want your reader to* *worry about.* For example, *The Healing*'s story question is, "Can Emmett Lee Westbrook ever reconcile with his children and learn to be a father?" This is the conflict from which the whole story unravels. So to immediately capture the viewer, it is introduced on page one of the script, Act One, Scene One. From the start, the audience is given a clear question or problem to worry about. If your story's question is incomprehensible to your viewers, then you probably haven't defined what the conflict of your story really is. And if you haven't given your audience anything to worry about, chances are, they won't! Your play's conflict may take place between two main characters (man against man), between a character and his surroundings (man against nature), or from within just one character (man against himself).

Man against God is also a good source of conflict—and one of the most intense. So stop right now and give your conflict precise definition in the form of a question. (One hint is that it may directly include your main character. After establishing a conflict, feel free to create many smaller conflicts to keep your audience guessing. These series of panic-relief episodes will propel your plot as your viewers wait to have the main conflict resolved.)

Resolution(s). The next natural progression is to now answer the question you first asked at the your story's beginning; by the way, of all the areas of flexibility given to a playwright during creation, this is not one of them! You must answer the story question and resolve the conflict. We've all seen a movie or two whose ending left us feeling cheated or stunned at its lack of completion. In the same way your audience will desire to have all loose ends "tied up" after their two-act journey with your relatable characters.

In answering the question for *The Healing*, we find the answer is, "Yes. Emmett can reconcile with his children, although it takes the impending death of his youngest daughter, Annie, to learn how to be a father, as he is left to care for her young daughter, Emma Lee." Before you begin writing, work out your play's conflicts and their resolutions. Be careful not to resolve them too quickly. For instance, if Emmett had reconciled with his children in Act I, what more could happen during Act II? Not much, since the main conflict would be resolved. Resolutions are best placed near the play's end, again, to keep your audience's attention.

Yawless Plot. As promised, plot will be discussed in this section. So far, you have a story idea (or a glimmer of one), your characters, their conflicts, and their resolutions. Plot is the series of events that moves your story through its conflict, its climax, and its resolution. In short, it's the progression of your story's action. (In filling the gap between the story question and the story answer of *The Healing*, introducing new characters, circumstances, and conflicts were necessary. These links, all chained together, are the plot.) However, "yawless" is the key word to this segment. Webster's defines *yaw* as (1) *to deviate from the intended course,* something you don't want your plot to do! So keep yourself in check along the writing process. For a simple illustration, let's say your story conflict is at #1 and the resolution is at #10. Then the natural progression, or plot, would be to count from 1 to 10, without pausing to add more impressive numbers such as 100 or 1,000. Do whatever it takes to get to 10, *but get there!* Don't take detours that don't interest your audience. A yawless plot is a crowd-pleaser!

Life-like Dialogue If storyline, plot, and theme are the ingredients of your play and your characters are preparing them, then surely your dialogue is the tray on which the whole feast will be served! Well-written words spoken by your story's characters will sink deeply into your viewers' minds and will be the cause of them remembering your play's many poignant moments. If your characters are "real," then so will be their conversations. This means they speak exactly as you would, using expressions, slang, and sometimes even speaking in incomplete sentences in order to stress certain emotions. The two most important rules to remember when writing dialogue are: (1) Let your characters do the talking, and (2) Allow only life-like dialogue and realistic conversations to occur. If you'll simply follow rule #1, rule #2 will happen all by itself. Really.

For instance, you are familiar with the biblical characters of Jesus Christ and Judas Iscariot, their conflict, and Christ's eventual resolution through the cross. We even have recorded for us some of their dialogue. But let's change the setting and place these two men in a modern-day setting somewhere near your town. What would they say to each other? You may initially predict that the change in setting would alter their conversation, but you can be sure that it would not. These two personalities are so well-defined that there is no doubt what they would *have* to say to each other. We would want Jesus to ask Judas, "Why did you betray Me and help cause My crucifixion?" But Jesus would be more likely to open His arms in forgiveness to Judas, assuring him that the crucifixion was God's plan and God's will to bring all of mankind into forgiveness and eternal security.

Judas, by nature, would struggle with forgiving himself, but might find peace in the fact that Christ still loved him.

Of course, these two biblical characters were real, living, breathing persons, and your fictional characters are not. Nonetheless, there is no reason why you can't become just as familiar with your characters and learn their natures so well, that their conversations will naturally flow from their own mouths. Pause briefly now to let two of your most well-defined characters speak to each other. Off the record, of course!

Inherent Theme Your theme is the main idea behind your entire story. It is the internal, elemental message that you want your audience to remember. Again, *The Healing* takes its characters through many emotional upheavals: the stress felt whenever Emmett's children visit; the disappointment Emmett displays at learning his granddaughter, Emma, is deaf; the flashback scenes that reveal the struggle surrounding the death of Emmett's wife to Huntington's Disease; the family's discovery that their youngest sister, Annie, has inherited the deadly Huntington's gene; and their urgent prayers for her healing; the final climax before Annie's death, between Annie and her father, as they both receive a much-needed emotional healing. Of all these moments, it is doubtful that those who have seen the play remember all the characters, their names, and their dilemmas. What they do remember of the play is its inherent theme: *a moving testimony of one family's miracle with the added reminder that to limit God is to deprive ourselves of the higher healing that rests just within our reach.* Before you continue, consider what the theme of your story is. Remember, storyline, plot, and theme differ greatly:

IF *STORYLINE* IS WHAT YOU BEGIN WITH,
AND *PLOT* IS WHAT YOU BUILD WITH,
THEN, *THEME* IS WHAT VIEWERS ARE LEFT WITH.

Natural Progressions. In the sport of long-distance running, pacing yourself is essential to finishing a race. If you want to do more than just finish, you must set a fast, yet comfortable, pace for each mile, and then adhere to it rigidly in order to endure the race and complete it at your expected time.

Likewise, pacing your plot is essential to good writing. As discussed in the resolutions segments, to introduce an answer to your story question too soon in the story leaves the audience with nothing to worry about for the rest of the play. Since keeping their interest is your goal, plan your dramatic action at a comfortable pace.

(1) Introduction of characters and main characters

(2) Introduction of conflict (and mini-conflicts)

(3) Introducing the opposing forces of your conflict(s), (man against man, man against nature, man against himself, man against God)

(4) Introduction of climax or major confrontation between your play's conflicting forces

(5) Final resolution, or the answer to your story problem or question

(6) The play's end

Although a rigid writing format is both unnecessary and restrictive for the creative writer, numbering your scenes and outlining their objectives will help you learn to pace your dramatic action. For an example of this, refer to the scene breakdown for *The Healing* at the end of this section. (Never begin writing with a story idea that hasn't been mapped out. Your action will be noticeably sluggish in some spots and too rushed in others.)

Plan approximately six scenes for each act you have scheduled to write. If you are planning a two-act play, you'll be working with twelve scenes. If you wish to write a one-act play, only six scenes will be necessary. The six progressions listed previously would be easily placed within a one-act play. Simply introduce your main characters and conflict between scenes one and two. Use your middle scenes for your mini-confrontations and play's body. Then, bring in major climax and resolutions in scenes five and six.

A two-act play is not measured quite the same because of the intermission between Acts I and II. Of course, you know that you'll want your play's main characters and conflicts introduced by Act I, Scenes One and Two. And again your climax and resolution should come at the end of Act II, right before the end of the play. So basically, you have four scenes in Act I (just before intermission) and four scenes in Act II (just after intermission) to introduce many minor characters whose mini-conflicts or mini-resolutions tie in and add to your main character's frustrations. So, if you plan—let's say—eight mini-confrontations and mini-conflicts that feed into or add a new twist to your main conflict, then pace yourself during these eight scenes and add one mini-conflict per scene. Skillfully build your tension to a point that your audience will be begging for the major climax and resolution!

What's even more important to pacing your action is keeping your audience's interest during the intermission by having planned a cliffhanger or perhaps a new conflict at the end of Act I. (For examples of Act I endings, read *The Inçentive* and *The Healing*.) By ending Act I with a surprising high-note (some sort of comic or tragic action, or even symbolism), your viewers will be so anxious for Act II to start that they won't even want an intermission!

As suggested, read *The Healing* and *The Inçentive*. The following is a scene-by-scene breakdown of the six necessary story progressions listed before. Next, map out the scene breakdown for your own storyline.

The Healing — ACT ONE

Scene 1—Emmett and Dory introduced. Conflict of the tension over Emmett's adult children introduced. Grace's death discussed. History information revealed through a flashback scene.

Scene 2—Dory schemes to invite the children for dinner against Emmett's wishes. Millie enters and announces her pregnancy. Dory and Millie chat, revealing more family history to the audience. Annie is discussed.

Scene 3—Ethan enters. Ethan, Millie, and Dory reveal even deeper family history, ending the scene with a flashback of Grace and her fatal disease.

Scene 4—Emmett discovers his children have come home, and he is angry, yet reserved.

Scene 5—Annie enters with her deaf daughter, Emma, having been away for five years. Claudia, Emmett's outspoken cousin, arrives with them, and the three of them take Emmett by surprise. He is angry at their presence and at Dory's scheming. Emmett explodes at the family dinner and exits. Claudia and Dory are at odds with each other.

Scene 6—Family continues eating without Emmett. Claudia is furious as Emmett's children defend him out of fear. They plan to confront Emmett during a family discussion. Annie reveals why she's stayed away for five years. In a flashback scene between a very young Claudia and young Grace, the audience learns why Claudia chose stardom over motherhood. Act I closes with Claudia rocking Emma to sleep, revealing signs of regret and sorrow over her life's choices.

ACT TWO

Scene 1—Emmett has skipped the planned family discussion. Dory is angry and ties him to a chair to speak her mind. Dory and Claudia find common ground for a friendship.

Scene 2—Annie enters and Claudia worries over Annie's ill health. (Her symptoms are those of the disease that killed her mother. Claudia doesn't recognize them, but the audience will.)

Scene 3—Ethan decides Annie's illness needs investigation and soon discovers that she indeed has the deadly symptoms of HD. A chilling flashback scene of the young Westbrook family at the funeral of their mother is seen. Ethan later informs Millie of Annie's symptoms.

Scene 4—The family waits as Dr. Grayson examines Annie upstairs. All are present except Emmett, as her disease is confirmed.

Scene 5—Emmett enters. Millie and Ethan tell him the news, but he does not respond. Annie enters and remains onstage alone with Emmett. Climax occurs through a confrontation. Reconciliation occurs.

Scene 6—Next morning the family tries to celebrate Christmas despite the news they've received. Emmett enters, a changed man from the emotional healing he's had. Annie is said to be in good spirits, despite her nearing death. The family is at total peace as Christmas carolers visit their door. All exit except Emmett as he realizes Emma hasn't heard the beautiful music. Seeing her need, he asks her to come stay with him, and she accepts. Emmett is given a second chance at fatherhood.

Evolution of Characters. The previous chart is the best way to see how characters evolve throughout a play. The conflict you introduce must touch each of your characters' lives and change them in some way. Of course, never candy-coat your endings and write unbelievable resolutions to your stories. Don't cheat your audience out of realistic solutions to the realistic problems they have watched your characters struggle through. If you do, your viewers will find no answer for themselves, and your play will have served no educational purpose. *The Healing* does end with the entire family at peace, so is this an unrealistic ending? No, because Annie will indeed die soon enough. Perhaps an unrealistic ending here would be to add to the emotional and spiritual healings that God granted a total physical healing for both Annie and Emma. (Unrealistic not because God isn't capable of such wonder, but because He chose to deliver a different healing to the Westbrooks.) Without any doubt, the exclusions of these physical ailments from these characters' lives would have resulted in the Westbrooks never receiving the emotional healing they needed so much more.

As you have worked your way through piecing together a good *storyline*, stop now and ask yourself the following questions about the evolutions or transformations your characters have made:

1. ARE THEY CLEAR?
2. ARE THEY REALISTIC? (No fairytale endings!)
3. WHAT WILL MY AUDIENCE LEARN FROM THEM?

PICK UP YOUR PEN! If you have in your mind a Setting, Timeless Characters, Obstacles, Resolutions, Yawless Plot, Life-like Dialogue, an Inherent Theme, Natural Progressions, and Evolution of Your Characters, then your storyline is ready! Congratulations on being three-fourths of the way through with your play *before* you've even begun writing! The time-saving *storyline* preparations you have made will save you from writing several rough drafts, because you know exactly where you are headed and the path you must take to get there. Find help labeling your storyline (comedy, drama, or melodrama) in the glossary at the end of this book. Also, your play should have a title before you begin writing your dialogue, and it should serve as a "quick commercial" for the contents of the storyline.

By now, your objectives and your characters are so clear in your mind that the dialogue, the actual writing of the play, will flow faster than you can pen it! Nonetheless, find a speedy pen and try to keep up with yourself. Good luck!

4

Casting a Play

Whether you have written your own play, or selected an existing one, you are now ready to begin casting. Casting a play is nothing more than filling each character role you have available with the most suitable actor in your drama troupe. It's not difficult, but it's no piece of cake either. Sometimes you won't have enough actors available to fill all your play's roles, and at other times you'll audition twice as many actors as you actually need. Remember, though, that when the latter happens, a place for most everyone can be found on a much-needed technical or production crew. In this chapter we'll pay close attention to the auditioning process, selecting production and technical help, and organizational meetings. Also, since this manual's majority readers are church dinner theatre organizers, helpful hints will be given on avoiding competition within the church and using everyone who auditions for your play.

The Audition

Ever seen *A Chorus Line*? Grueling. Of course, it very realistically depicts the ups and downs of the auditioning process. And for the actor who is chosen, a real high is achieved from knowing he or she has "beaten" all the other actors who auditioned for that role. In secular theatre, this attitude is fed and even rewarded. But, in the church, it has no place. The auditioning process is an exciting part of the professional actor's life because his livelihood depends on it. But while most of the people who audition alongside of him in a secular production will be total strangers, those who audition alongside of him in a church production will not be. They are his friends. And long after the audition is over, he must continue to see these people, serve on church committees with them, and even worship with them. For this reason, the church dinner theatre director must manage to keep competition and rivalry out of its auditions and away from his drama troupes.

By now, you are wondering how an audition with no competitive edge can be an audition at all! The truth is that your audition must have a competitive edge for it to be successful, but your actors must *not* have a competitive spirit or they won't *feel* successful. How is all this accomplished? Very, very easily.

1. First, hold your auditions on two separate days, one week apart, to ensure that everyone who wants to attend can work it into their schedules. Allow two to three hours for each of these days.

2. Advertise the auditions well in your newsletters, bulletins, or during your meetings and refer to the auditions as "tryouts." Through word of mouth, personally invite people to the tryouts, assuring them that professional actors are not necessary to make a good production!

3. On the first day you meet, the director should request the following information from everyone who attends:

NAME - AGE - ADDRESS - PHONE NUMBER (WORK AND HOME), PREFERENCE: CAST OR CREW, CONFLICTS DURING SCHEDULED REHEARSAL TIMES, HOBBIES, CLOTHES SIZE, HEIGHT, WEIGHT, ETC.

4. Next, distribute a list of technical and production crews and ask everyone present to sign their name by any field that interests them. This way, if they do not get a speaking role, they can be most appropriately directed to the crew on which they will most enjoy. A detailed description of each crew is outlined in Chapter 7: Technical Techniques.

5. Next, have enough copies of your script for each character role and simply begin discussing the play and its characters. Then begin reading through the play, alternating roles and seeing which actors best fit all the parts. (The director should make notes on the back of the actor-info sheets collected above.)

6. Eliminate "cattle call" auditions and don't require your actors to come with prepared monologues. Cutting straight to the play by having a casual "cold reading" will not only relax your actors and let them shine, but it will also take the pressure off the director in casting. Here, the auditions are motivated by the others' reading, and are also allowed to see for themselves who is really best for each role.

7. Give everyone a date by which they will be called and notified of the role they will fill. Assure them that they all will be given a role, either in the cast or the crew, and that both are vital to a performance.

Ask everyone to hold open the first scheduled rehearsal date so they can return and pick up a script and a copy of the entire season's rehearsal schedule. (The cast will attend all rehearsals, whereas the crew will be pulled in during the last few weeks of production. See Chapter 6 for rehearsal coordination.)

By the time you have gone through these seven steps, on two different days, you will have a good indication of which actors will best fill all the roles for your play. The technical/production crew sheet you distributed will also have many of its committees filled. Next all you'll have to do is fill in the blanks, like finding extra people to serve on those crews that no one signed up for, or auditioning some people privately to fill those unspoken-for roles. Don't despair if you have more "blanks" than you do "filled roles" on your first couple of productions. As your dinner-theatre popularity increases, so will the number of people who want to help.

Sometimes, several competent actors will read for the same role, leaving the director with a tough decision to make. If this happens in your case, then narrow down the process by studying the actor information sheets. Which one of the actors can be at *all* rehearsals? This person is your surest bet, since a rehearsal with even one actor absent can slow down the entire operation. If after looking over their actor information sheets, your selection is still not made easy, then consider the physical attributes of the character in question. Which actor best fits that description or build? These questions should be considered whenever casting takes place.

Technical and Production Crews

The following is a list of various committees and crews that will need filling for a successful dinner-theatre production:

Director / Producer / House Affairs Coordinator / Creative Affairs Coordinator / Lighting Foreman / Sound Foreman / Additional Technical Support Helpers / Stage Manager / Set Design and Coordinator / Properties Manager / Prop Assistants / Makeup and Hair Specialists / Set Foreman / Set or Scenery Builders / House Managers / Ushers / Publicity Coordinators / Ticket Reservationists / Children's Backstage Assistance / Kitchen Managers / Costume Designer / Program Flyer Printing / Video Editing (if you film the production)

As you can see, these parts greatly outnumber the parts in your average-size cast. So finding the right person for each committee is just as vital as casting your play's speaking roles. (Chapter 7: Technical Techniques is devoted to describing the functions of each of these roles.)

Organizational Meetings

By your first rehearsal, your Lighting Foreman, Sound Foreman, Stage Manager, and Prop Manager should all have copies of the script you are performing. As stated, you'll be working with the cast more at first than you will with the crews. So, an early technical/production meeting will be needed to organize the various crew managers and to motivate them to start planning for their individual areas of responsibilities. Attending the first technical/production meeting should be your Light Foreman, Sound Foreman, Technical Coordinator, House Coordinator, Creative Affairs Coordinator, Costumer, Musical Coordinator, Stage Manager, Prop Manager, and Set Designer. Listen to one another's ideas, allowing the Director to make all the final decisions.

After casting all technical/production crews, keep in touch with the crews until it is time for them to begin attending practices. As for the actors, they too will be hard at work, studying their characters and learning their lines. If every person involved will do his or her job with diligence, the production will benefit from it and your dinner theatre will be a raving success!

5

The Director's Chair

The title "Director" might seem to some like an impressively illustrious position. However, anyone who has ever sat in the director's chair knows that it is often the most uncomfortable seat in the house. In fact, the energy and endurance it takes to direct your production will leave you asking why director's chairs were ever invented in the first place, as you will rarely find yourself sitting down. However, there are few greater rewards than a production will done, and you as the director are the pivotal influence which can insure a successful dinner theatre for you and your drama troupe.

Essentially this entire book is written as a director's manual, but this chapter especially is dedicated to the pursuit of skillful direction and to the search for those who are waiting to learn how. A dinner-theatre director's job differs slightly from that of a regular director. He or she not only directs the actors in the play, but is also responsible for coordinating and managing all the committees necessary to cater and prepare for such a large event.

Logically, two people should share this job—one person to direct the dinner portion of dinner theatre and one person to direct the actual theatre portion. However, not only is having two directors very confusing, but the two jobs are so deeply intertwined as to create the perfectly matched dinner-theatre mood, that from these two directors would be required extraordinary communication and endless meeting with each other. Ideally, one person should direct the play and oversee its multiple dinner-theatre committees, which should each then have a manager. This way, the managers are covering ground that the director could never manage alone, while their efforts will serve as an active voice throughout the entire shaping of the play itself. First things first, of course. The whole process does begin with the selection of the play, which naturally is the director's first job.

1. Choosing a play—This can appear to be the most time-consuming part of the directing process, but don't become discouraged. Remember to think of your audience long before you select a play and to ask yourself what they'll want or need to see. Other factors such as your actors, rehearsal time, and available rehearsal and performance space also play a large role in this decision. Are you hoping to entertain or educate your audience? Remember that both can be effectively achieved by simply finding the right play. Are you looking for a comedy or a drama? Perhaps you are only planning an annual holiday dinner theatre, in which case you can begin searching directly for Easter or Christmas plays. Don't forget the "Choosing a Play" quiz in Chapter 2. The quiz and the entire chapter will help you decide what type of play best suits your drama troupe's needs. Once you decide, shop around in bookstores, libraries, church libraries, and Christian bookstores, and especially in dramatic publishing house catalogues.

2. Casting the play—Again, this is an important part of the director's task and an entire chapter of this book, Chapter 4, is designed to help make auditions more natural and less competitive, especially within the church dinner theatre. Refer to the seven points listed in Chapter 4 for assistance in casting your play. The "unveiling" and reading of the selected play, plus filling all its character roles, can be the most charging and least timely positions that the director will hold, if he or she has organized and planned ahead. Step 3 will help you start doing just that.

3. Reading and rereading the selected play—Once your play has been selected, you are ready to begin dissecting it. Never direct before you dissect! Start by reading the play through once for an overview of the story without forming any opinions. Later, read it again, making careful notes on the inherent theme that the playwright is striving to communicate.

Next, discover the progression of your plot by mapping out each scene on a separate sheet of paper and listing the objectives, goals, and moods for each scene. For instance, if in Scene 2 your main character enters and is faced with the major struggle of the play, then your list would state: "Act I, Scene 2 - Main character introduced; conflict established; mood: discouraging and solemn." You might even note which character is responsible for initiating and communicating this mood to the audience, and write his or her name next to the mood. By documenting your mood changes from scene to scene, you and your actors will be more apt to convey them.

Share this list with your actors during your tablework rehearsals to help them in their deliveries. Also allow your technical crews to view copies of the list at your first production meeting. Pay close attention to any suggestions they have that would enhance each scene's mood. Finally, examine each character thoroughly. What does this character add each time he or she is on stage? Never expect your actors to get to know their characters unless you too have first become mindfully acquainted with them.

4. Now that you have cast your play and have become keenly aware of its scenes, characters, and moods, you can begin preblocking its movement or choreography. By now, you should have designed your set, or met with your set designer and discussed your set's layout. For example, if your play occurs in someone's living room, you must first decide where that person's sofa is before you can have him advance to that location to sit on it.

As the director, you probably have the best ideas about your script's needs for set design. With you as the set designer, you can easily pre-block the play, allowing a set construction foreman or scenery manager to actually build the set you design. Also, a set-donation coordinator should be named to begin collecting the furniture and decorations you will need to make your set a "home." Once your set design is on paper, distribute copies of your technical and production crews to assist them in their tasks of placing lights and planting hidden microphones (if your performance area requires this).

With all this in place, pre-blocking your actor's stage movements can occur. Pre-blocking is always tentative, of course, since the actual blocking rehearsals will best determine which stage movements look best and feel most natural to your actors. (Considering the actors' natural impulses and urges is worthwhile to you as the director, although you are responsible for seeing to it that they are effective and consistent to the mood of each scene. To illustrate, if in a heartbreaking scene your actor decides his character would most likely whisper his last few lines while kneeling, consider and even allow him to try this. However, do not allow this blocking to remain if you have walked the performance area during his attempt and been unable to hear or see him deliver these vital lines.) Pre-blocking your script before the actual blocking rehearsals truly expedites the tedious task of blocking. At times, your actors may feel that "blocking rehearsals" are full of many stops and starts. They are, of course, to the betterment of the production, but pre-blocking eliminates many of those numerous interruptions.

The set design, the script, and some imaginative visualization is all the director needs when pre-blocking. If you find that remembering where you've previously placed each actor is too difficult, then simply cut out small pieces of colored construction paper with your cast members' names on them and actually move them around your set design sheet as you pre-block. With your play tentatively blocked, you are almost ready to begin rehearsing it. So turn your efforts now toward making the most of each practice, and organize your rehearsals before they've even begun.

5. Organizing Rehearsal Time—A complete rehearsal format is located in the next chapter, Practice Makes Perfect . . . or Does It? There you will learn how a drama team can maximize every rehearsal by following a detailed rehearsal schedule. You, as the director, are responsible for compiling that schedule (keeping your actor's schedules in mind as much as possible), and for seeing to it that your actors follow it. Each actor should receive a copy of this schedule and should be able to ascertain from it which rehearsals they are required to attend. If your cast members see you have organized well and are maximizing their personal time, they will be more likely to attend their required rehearsals and put forth their absolute best.

6. Conducting rehearsals—This area may have been your original impression of a director's *real* job. By now, you may have guessed that a dinner theatre director's job description is infinite! Still, this one task of shaping your dinner theatre's play is truly the most exhilarating, as well as the most absorbing. If you have familiarized yourself with the play, pre-blocked it, and organized your rehearsal times beforehand, you will be afforded the wonderful experience of spending each rehearsal fully engrossed in your actors and in keeping them on the right course.

Remember that rehearsals should be equally as fulfilling for your actors, and that their ideas and needs for experimentation are fully as important as yours. Your job is not to dominate them, but to serve them, helping them in their roles and guiding them gently toward the play's main goal. Keep in mind that once you demand respect, you've lost it and that unless the rehearsals remain pleasant for everyone, your first dinner-theatre production may well be your last.

7. Ministering to your cast as a mediator and a disciplinarian—This segment has in mind the director who has truly tried to maintain harmony both within and with all the cast members but is experiencing discouragement despite his or her efforts. Few people will be able to understand the

extreme pressure you are under during the many weeks of rehearsing the production. The ones who do understand this stress will become your greatest sources of encouragement and emotional nourishment. Remember that no one is perfect, not even you, and that you must always keep yourself in check. In the church environment, this must undoubtedly be your most crucial commitment to your cast. That, plus remembering that they are not *your* cast. You are merely overseeing a group of people, often many people, who are all striving to fulfill their areas of service to God. Again, your service is to your actors, as well as to your Heavenly Father, and He will reward and recognize your honest efforts even if they do not.

Creative people are very sensitive by nature, or they would be unable to be so creative! They are very in-touch with their feelings, which in turn enables them to feel things more quickly and more deeply than the average person, thus feeding the creative process. Naturally, then, a creative person has a tendency to have his or her feelings hurt more quickly than the average person. Assemble a large group of creative people for a series of long rehearsals, and it is inevitable, therefore, that you will experience some turbulent times.

If two of your cast members are noticeably at odds with each other, then consider moving them to another position within the cast so they will not have to work so closely together. However, not only is this impossible if you are close to your performance, but sweeping any conflict under the carpet is unhealthy as well as unbiblical. If it is too late in rehearsals to switch any roles, and if you feel close enough to both parties to approach them, then do so. Prayerfully! Let them do most of the talking and think of what is best for their friendship, not for the play. Naturally, if the conflict is removed and they forgive each other, then the play will improve along with their friendship. If however, in a Christian dinner-theatre the problem is between you (the director) and a cast member, then the obligation for reconciliation is up to you. Why? Because your Christian brother or sister will expect it from you, and as a responsible Christian it is your duty. The other party involved is not exempt from initiating reconciliation, but since you are the director, he or she may wait for you to attempt peace first. Of course, this is impossible if you do not even realize that anyone is angry with you! In such a case, the dinner theatre member who has a complaint against you must inform you before they can expect you to apologize or alter your behavior. This is not just some sort of courtesy. It is a biblical commandment found in Matthew 18:15-16:

Moreover if your brother sins against you, go and tell him his fault between you and him alone. If he hears you, you have gained your brother. But if he will not hear you, take with you one or two more, that by the mouth of two or three witnesses every word may be established.

Likewise, as the director, communicate privately with each cast member often and express any problems you may feel he or she has posed—not as his or her director, but as a friend. Remember, the mature Christian has no need for grudges, and neither does the mature director.

8. Overseeing all the dinner theatre committees—In any dinner theatre production, there are anywhere from twenty to thirty committee or crews, each with a separate manager. Most committees are made up of only one person, the manager, as in the case of stage management. Some committees require little effort, and so one person may be able to effectively manage two different crews. For instance, on the evenings of your performances your house managers are in charge of greeting the guests and overseeing the ushers who seat each visitor. House management and ushering are really two different crews, but there is no reason why a responsible house manager cannot slip away now and again to help the ushers get everyone seated. Of course, make sure that the main entrance is never left unattended, or someone without a ticket may slip in and claim a taken seat!

Nonetheless, regardless of how many managers you end up with, you are responsible for communicating to each of them his or her exact job description and for aiding that manager in clearly understanding the deadlines that committee faces. Choose managers that will keep in contact with you, since there is no way you can be expected to call twenty to thirty people each week to make sure they are doing their jobs. As the dinner theatre director, if you feel that directing the actual play is all you can handle, then consider finding a producer or another director to oversee all the dinner theatre committees. However, as stated at the start of the chapter, this will actually be more difficult at times, since you as the director will lose all creative control over much of the dinner theatre-environment.

The play's mood should govern all aspects of the meal, the environment, the music, and even the table centerpieces. Since you as the director will be most familiar with the play's mood, you are the logical person to oversee all the committees, allowing each committee's manager to carry out all necessary duties. Some areas of dinner theatre need only a one-time coordination and not a full-time committee. (A good example of this is finding a photographer to come to one of your rehearsals two weeks before the performances and take publicity shots during an entire run-thru of the play. These pictures are displayed locally as inexpensive advertisement, and most photographers will donate a few hours of their time to your production, especially if it is a church production. You may wish to call on a church member who is a photographer. This photographer is easily coordinated, so you as the director can easily make that phone call and eliminate the need for an entirely separate committee or manager for this. Likewise, working with a caterer can be just as easy, since all that is required is scheduling their services far in advance and keeping in touch with them to confirm your planned menu as the performances near.) The director can easily handle these few phone calls, especially if the same familiar caterer is used from year to year. However, if during your first season you find yourself spending too much precious time locating a caterer, then feel free to ask for help, and appoint a catering coordinator to find the most appropriate caterer to fit your production and your budget.

9. Serving your cast—It is worth repeating that your job as a director is not to dominate the cast and crew, but to serve them. How can you serve them? Help the actors find their ways. Help your props manager know exactly what props you have in mind. Help the lighting and sound foremen by being patient as they strive to heighten each scene's mood with their special effects. Help your costume designer visualize each character's apparel. And most importantly, help yourself by allowing each of them to do his or her job.

10. Praying for your cast—In the Christian dinner-theatre environment, this is a must. Begin praying for the cast before there is one, just following the selection of a play. Prayerfully place each person in the best role or on a crew that best suits him or her. Prepare yourself spiritually before each rehearsal with a quiet time and some time in God's Word. Open and close each rehearsal with prayer, asking various cast members to lead the group. Schedule private meetings with all the individual cast members before opening night and speak with them about their character questions, personal lives, and any needs for prayer they may have. These brief meetings and private prayer times take only about five minutes and can be scheduled before or after any rehearsal. Or if you sense that one of the cast members needs an extra lift, take them out for coffee, hold your brief-

meeting, and then close by praying for them. Take care of your cast. If they sense your care and appreciation, it will be difficult for them ever to doubt your motives.

On a final note, think long and hard before you agree ever to sit in the director's chair. Remember it is less like a recliner and more like a wooden stool that you must perch on, stand behind, and sometimes kneel beside in prayer. You will need to have the aptitude to begin a work and the competence to see it through. Organizational skills will be needed to avoid any last-minute, feverish rushes. You will serve as a compass for your actors and as a hub for your technical/production crews. Do you possess forbearance? Composure? Creativity? Endurance? Self-control? Tolerance? Patience? Good. No one person does! However, if you are willing to learn and eager to try, then you might just discover that the director's chair doesn't have to be the most uncomfortable seat in the house. In fact, it might just be the best.

6

Practice Makes Perfect . . . Or Does It?

Rehearsals

It's been said that "practice makes perfect," and, of course, rehearsals *are* a form of practice. So, do rehearsals make for a perfect performance? Hardly. Be that as it may, if you do not ever strive for perfection, you are sure never to even come close to it.

So then, what is a rehearsal? In *Webster's Dictionary*, the word "rehearse" falls somewhere in between rehash and reinforce, which is quite appropriate. In fact, all the surrounding words begin with "re," which means "repetition of a previous action." To reheat means to heat again. To recount means to count again. So what are we doing when we rehearse?

> Hearse (hurs)—A vehicle for conveying a dead body to a cemetery

Surely not! On the other hand, perhaps this is where the expression "we're beating a dead horse" comes from after a long and grueling rehearsal. Here is the real definition of rehearse:

1. v. to practice in preparation for a public performance.
2. to perfect, or cause to perfect (an action) by repetition.

Now that you know what a rehearsal *is*, let's discuss how to make the most of one. Like a teacher in a classroom, the director is to be in charge of the rehearsal period. Firmly, but gently, he or she is to have organized the rehearsal time, and then must steadily keep it on track. (See Chapter 5, segments 5 and 6.) This means beginning on time. Of course, never pressure everyone to rush into his or her spot, or the result of this will be a poor performance during rehearsal. Besides, if your rehearsal begins at 6:30 p.m. you can be sure that the majority of the cast will arrive no sooner than 6:30. This means you must first set and prepare your stage as they arrive to lend you a hand, so your actual rehearsal may not begin until somewhere between 6:45 and 7. In short, your actual "rehearsing" may not begin as soon as everyone enters, but see to it that preparations for it do (stage set-up, actor warm-ups, prayer time, etc.). Also, never wait on each actor to be present before beginning your stage rehearsing, even if you are certain that the one who is late is on his or her way. This is unfair to those who were punctual. If a rehearsal begins late, it is most likely to end late, all because of those few tardy members. Plus, when late cast members arrive and find you already rehearsing, they are sure to be punctual, if not early, to the next rehearsal. In the church dinner theatre, it is helpful to remember that most of the actors are amateurs. They have jobs, church activities, families, and children to work around, and the dinner theatre production will not be their most important priority. That's not to say that discipline and commitment cannot be expected from them, because it should be if they have decided to involve themselves. The director will have the responsibility of casting only those people who can attend rehearsals and be punctual. Otherwise, it is also his or her responsibility to speak to any member who is bringing difficulty to the rehearsal schedule, or to find a replacement for that role. This is not always a pleasant task, but if not done, then the rest of the cast and their hard work will be jeopardized.

Prompt beginnings and endings are one way to show the cast you care about their time. Another way is to maximize their time by having them attend only those rehearsals at which they are needed. Before fully exploring how an actor's time can be maximized, or made the most of, we'll create a mock-rehearsal schedule for a full two-act play, and then study it carefully. Let's first decide how many total rehearsal hours you need and when to schedule each rehearsal period.

Total Rehearsal Hours Needed

A good rule for rehearsal time is to plan fifteen hours of rehearsal time for each thirty minutes of performance time. If you are performing a one-act play of one hour in length, then plan on approximately thirty hours of rehearsal time. (If your rehearsals last three hours, plan ten rehearsals. If they last two hours, plan for fifteen meetings.) If you are performing a two-act play of approximately one hour and thirty minutes in length, then count on scheduling forty-five hours of rehearsal time. (That's twenty-three rehearsals at two hours each, or fifteen rehearsals at three hours each.)

Scheduling Rehearsals & Performances

Whatever the amount of total rehearsal hours you need, begin now to schedule them over a period of time which is comfortable for your actors. Of course, it's easier to find actors to work their schedules into the one you have planned, than it is to plan a schedule based around twenty different people's needs. So begin by suggesting the following schedule techniques to the cast:

1. Rehearse over a period of two full months with performance dates at the end of the second month or at the very beginning of the third month. (For example, rehearse in July and August and perform at the very end of August or at the beginning of September.)

2. For your first month of rehearsals, meet only on Saturdays to study the play's characters and block the play's movements. Set rehearsal times for three hours.

3. Beginning the second month, continue to meet on Saturdays as well as adding two weeknight rehearsals. Keep rehearsals at three hours each.

4. The week of your performances (Saturdays are best for Opening Night), hold your regular two weekly rehearsals and add a Friday-night dress rehearsal the night before your play opens. (Let the cast and crew know this will probably be a late night in case you need to rehearse the play twice.) As mentioned, try to schedule your Opening Night for a Saturday night. Not only does this work well for rehearsals, but Saturdays are always a popular "weekend night out," and ticket sales are always excellent. Depending on how much money you need to recoup for your dinner-theatre expenses, plan for at least two performances: a Saturday night and a Sunday matinee. (See Chapter 11, Budgeting and Publicity, for more scheduling suggestions.)

5. Depending on which months you rehearse and perform in, and on how the days of the week fall, you should have between fifty and sixty hours of total rehearsal time with this schedule. A full-length, two-act, 1½-2-hour play can be well-rehearsed using this format. If you are performing only a one-act, one-hour play and need less total rehearsal hours, then shorten your rehearsal time to two hours, but still hold your fifteen needed meetings over two months (15 meetings X 2 hours each = 30 hours total rehearsal time).

During these two months, two rehearsals a week for eight weeks would be ideal spacing. Primarily, two months is the minimum in which a dinner theatre can be produced. Always remember, even though the theatrical portion may be near completion, the many committees who plan the dinner, costumes, scenery, and lighting may not be.

Organizing Individual Rehearsal Periods

After figuring your total number of rehearsal hours needed and after deciding when your rehearsals and performances will be, then organize each individual rehearsal period. During a two to three hour rehearsal, four scenes can easily be practiced. This works out well if your two-act play has twelve scenes as do *The Incentive* and *The Healing*. Simply break the play into three sections of four scenes each and rehearse one of these sections each time you are together. Section one would be Act I, Scenes 1,2,3, and 4. Section two would be Act I, Scenes 5 and 6 plus Act II, Scenes 1 and 2. Section three would be Act II, Scenes 3,4,5, and 6.

Note on the following rehearsal schedule that during the second month of rehearsals, the cast meets three times a week, rehearsing one section of the play each time. This allows the entire play to be rehearsed by the week's end. This is an effective work schedule which benefits the play and also allows the actors to be present only when needed. As an example, if in the play a particular actor appears only in Act I, Scene 5 and in Act II, Scenes 1 and 2, then he would look on the rehearsal schedule and see that during the busy month of August, when the majority of the cast is meeting three times a week, he needs to be there only once a week, on Tuesdays. Only characters who are in all three sections of your play will need to be present at all rehearsals. Planning in this fashion will be greatly appreciated by your cast, and their work will reflect it.

Rehearsal Schedule

Saturday, July 6—Tablework and Character Analysis—Act I and Act II
Saturday, July 13—In-depth Character Analysis—Both Acts
Saturday, July 20—Block Act I, Scenes 1,2,3 & 4
Saturday July 27—Block Act I Scenes 5 & 6, Act II, Scenes 1 & 2
Thursday, August 1—Block Act II, Scenes 3,4,5 & 6
Saturday, August 3—Rehearse Act I, Scenes 1,2,3, & 4
Tuesday, August 6—Rehearse Act I, Scenes 5 & 6, Act II, Scenes 1 & 2
Thursday, August 8—Rehearse Act II, Scenes 3,4,5, & 6
Saturday, August 10—Rehearse Act I, Scenes 1,2,3, & 4
Tuesday, August 13—Rehearse Act I, Scenes 5 & 6, Act II, Scenes 1 & 2
Thursday, August 15—Rehearse Act II, Scenes 3,4,5, & 6
Saturday, August 17—BE OFF BOOK! Act I, Scenes 1,2,3, & 4

Tuesday, August 20—BE OFF BOOK! Act I, Scenes 5,6/Act II, Scenes 1,2

Thursday, August 22—BE OFF BOOK! Act II, Scenes 3,4,5, & 6

Saturday, August 24—FINAL POLISHING ACT I, Scenes 1,2,3, & 4

Tuesday, August 27—FINAL POLISHING ACT I, Sc. 5 & 6/ACT II, Sc. 1,2

Tuesday, August 29—FINAL POLISHING ACT II, Scenes 3,4,5, & 6

Saturday, August 31—EXTENSIVE WORK-ACT I, Sc. 1 & 6/ACT II, Sc. 1 & 6

Tuesday, September 3—WET TECH REHEARSAL—no costumes, but full run-thru!

Thursday, September 5—FULL DRESS REHEARSAL WITH LIGHTS, SOUND, & COSTUMES!

Friday, September 6—FULL DRESS WITH NO STOPPING—PLAN FOR A LATE NIGHT.

Saturday, September 7—PERFORMANCE, MAKEUP CALL AT   5:30/SHOW AT 7:00

Sunday, September 8—PERFORMANCE, MAKEUP CALL—10:45/SHOW AT 12:30 p.m.

Monday, September 9—PERFORMANCE, MAKEUP CALL 5:30/SHOW AT 7:00

REHEARSAL TIMES: ALL EVENING REHEARSALS (TUES./THURS.) ARE FROM 6:30-9:00 p.m. ALL SATURDAY REHEARSALS ARE FROM 2:00-4:00 p.m.

PLEASE BE **ON TIME** TO HELP WITH STAGE SET-UP AND THEN, BREAKDOWN.

BEGIN PRAYING *NOW* FOR THE CAST, CREWS, AND AUDIENCE!

Notice that the first two rehearsals are spent on character analysis. During these rehearsals, the cast is seated in a circle, and the play is read from beginning to end with the sole purpose of helping the actor discover each scene's mood and how his or her character contributes to it. These rehearsals are full of starts and stops, repeating certain lines until each actor has begun to "feel" his part. After those two rehearsals, the cast should be so involved with their characters and with the play that they are ready to "walk it." Blocking, or stage movement, can now begin. The director should have already tentatively pre-blocked the play and now simply leads the cast through each scene, telling them where to sit, when to rise, etc. The cast should have a pencil and script in hand on stage and should make careful notes on their movements, marking them in their scripts. Attendance at blocking rehearsals is mandatory, and after the entire play is choreographed, rehearsing can begin at the very next practice.

"Rehearsing" rehearsals take up the largest block of your overall schedule. Here, you reinforce blocking, help the actors become familiar with their set and props, and encourage them to learn their lines while making sure that with each rehearsal their characters become more defined. Somewhere during this portion of rehearsals, each cast member should turn in to the director his or her character biography sheet (detailed in Chapter 10, Acting). This sheet of in-depth character questions will stimulate thought in each actor's mind about who he or she is portraying. Those actors who truly study their characters will give the most notable performances.

After this amount of rehearsing, the play should be coming together quite nicely. The actors also should be ready to lay down their scripts. Many may have already done this, but as soon as everyone is "off book" the play can really make great strides in terms of dramatic expression. From this point on, request that your actors never take their scripts back on stage. Oh, they may stumble through one or two rehearsals and need line-assistance from the director, but don't worry. They won't be pleased with their own performances and before long, they'll no longer need prompting!

Your play is now looking more and more like a full-stage production as some of the technical crews begin to attend rehearsals and add their special touches. Props, scenery, and stage design are exciting the actors and enhancing their performances. Final polishing will happen naturally. During each scene of each rehearsal, the director should make detailed notes of that scene's good points and bad points. Technical crews should also be reminded during these rehearsals of the props or furniture the set is lacking. One special rehearsal should be for extensive work on the first and last scenes of each act. These are crucial scenes to the play, and close attention should be given to improving the pace of each of these four scenes. Your audience will be paying closer attention to these parts of the play, and you'll want to leave them with a good impression.

During the Wet-tech rehearsal, your lighting and sound crews must be present. The cast performs the entire play, with no costumes, while the lighting and sound foremen make final notes on their technical cues (phone rings, dimming lights, doorbells, etc.). This rehearsal should finalize and answer any questions the technical crew has regarding where lights should be hung or what hidden microphones will be needed. After the Wet-tech rehearsal, these major technical jobs can begin.

Two full-dress rehearsals are necessary before Opening Night. By the first one, lights should be hung, and all technical equipment, including any amplification needs, should be in place. In full costume, the cast performs the entire play for the first time with total technical enhancements. At the end of this rehearsal, the entire dinner theatre cast and crew assembles for the director's notes. Again, the director has watched with a close eye, and with a fine-tooth comb has documented everything about the play that needs praising or changing.

The next night, at the final dress rehearsal, the play is again performed, this time with no stopping. The actors must have one rehearsal where they never break character. Inform them ahead of time that if any actor misses a line during this rehearsal, he or she must keep going and learn on their own to save the scene without breaking character. If they do not exercise this at least once, they will be unable to do this during a live performance. Your final dress rehearsal may be a long one, requiring two run-thrus. The last time the play is rehearsed, the director should try to refrain from giving any "bad-director notes." Even if the play still needs a little work, at this point offering praise will do a lot more good than giving them too much to think about just before Opening Night.

The final preparation is blocking your curtain call. Your curtain call is when all the actors take their bows to music at the end of the performance. Starting with the most minor characters and ending with the main character of the production, the actors should file on stage. One by one, they take an individual bow at center stage, then find a place to sit or stand on the set. After the main character bows, the entire cast rises for an "all-company bow." Then they exit off-sage (starting with the main character and going through the cast) and form a reception line by the exit door. As the audience leaves, they are allowed a chance to visit with the cast. (This portion is always a real highlight of the performances, both for the cast and the audience!)

After the rehearsals studied in this chapter you should be able to answer the question, Practice makes perfect . . . or does it?" Most likely, your answer will be "no," but you won't be discouraged. On opening night, a feeling of intoxicating satisfaction will sweep over the entire cast and crew, leaving behind only the memories of the audience's laughter and tears.

Rehearse—2. to perfect, or cause to perfect (an action) by repetition

Always keep your Opening Night in mind, and remember this Webster's definition of rehearse at each and every discouraging rehearsal you might have. The point is: a perfect work is impossible, but "to perfect" your work is not.

7

Technical Techniques

And who will listen to you in this matter? For as his share is who goes down to the battle, so shall his share be who stays by the baggage; **they shall share and share alike**" (1 Sam. 30:24, author's boldface).

Never underestimate the importance of any technical crew to your dinner-theatre production. Depending on the size of your group, your play, and your performance area, you'll need anywhere from fifteen to thirty technical and production crews. Some crews will staff only one person, and others will need several more. But whatever the number of technical and production workers you end up with, you can be sure that they will hold within their hands the play you have painfully selected, cast, rehearsed, and essentially given birth to. Therefore, you may as well learn to think of these people as your delivery coaches! Not only do all of these people greatly outnumber your cast, but they have within their power the ability to make or break a show.

Consider exactly what would happen if, as an actor, you are on stage alone, having just finished a rather long, emotional speech. You pause, waiting for the sound of a ringing phone to interrupt the silence, break the mood, and give you motivation to rise and cross to the telephone. You wait. And wait. No ring. So, you panic. Of course, not half as much as the sound foreman does as he realizes his ringer has a short in it. Realizing the phone call is crucial to the scene, you decide to cross to the phone, pick it up, and call the party who was supposed to call you. Just as you do, however, that short in the ringer decides to behave, and there you stand, dialing a ringing phone.

Or even worse, imagine that your scenery-construction foreman has built an ornately beautiful staircase, and you are waiting offstage, preparing to make an angry entrance. Storming onto the set, you march down the stairs and are fully on the stage when you realize that the last piece of banister you gripped is still in your hand. The audience roars with laughter, you want to run back upstairs, and your poor scenery foreman has probably fled the building.

From personal experience, both of these scenarios are highly stressful and embarrassing to the actor on stage. Neither of the tragedies were his fault, yet he is the one left to recover the fumbled mood and save the scene. It should be noted that an unexpected short in a wire cannot be helped, but a simple hammer and a few nails could've prevented that last story. The first lesson to be learned here is that you should first staff your technical and production crews only with responsible people. And the second lesson? Pray that they can think *fast* on their feet!

Sound Needs: Again, the amount of dinner theatre crews you will need will depend on how much technical assistance your play needs. As a measure for you let's consider *The Healing*. It was first performed by the First Baptist Church of Donelson, Tennessee, Dinner Theatre and was staged in the church's Family Life Center. It is a standard gymnasium with a regulation-size basketball court, and each year we transform it into a beautiful dinner theatre. The FLC, with our thirty-five round tables and folding chairs has a seating capacity of 280 people. Even though the actors have to work very hard on projection in a gymnasium, 280 people inevitably absorb a lot of that projected sound. So, to improve audibility we use hanging shotgun microphones (a directional microphone useful in amplifying only your desired area). We then find inconspicuous locations to hide tiny lapel or clip-on microphones in central floral centerpieces or on desk tops, etc. Of course, a sure way for each actor to be heard is to have each wear a lapel microphone, but this is highly discouraged. Not only are they nearly $1,000 each, but the thought of each actor sounding so artificially amplified is very contradictory to the true-theatrical atmosphere. After all, do you roam about in *your* living room speaking into a micro-phone? Of course not, and if your actors do this in their living areas, it will seem equally as unnatural to your audience. *The Healing* also required hanging a shotgun microphone over the auxiliary stage used for the flashback scenes. Other than this, the only other sound effects were telephone rings.

Lighting Needs Special attention will be given here to lights because of their crucial importance to your production. If you are unfamiliar with the various types of lighting equipment, then talk with a knowledgeable light-ing engineer or ask questions of the numerous lighting consultants where lights can be rented. If your knowledge of lighting is limited, then renting may be best for you. Simply look in your local Yellow-Page directory under "Lighting Systems and Equipment." ("Lighting Consultants and Designers" may also have some stage equipment available.) Here you will find experienced technicians who know the answers to all of your questions. Even if you aren't sure what questions to ask, meet with them and describe to them your play and your budget. Their suggestions will be most helpful in determining what lights to rent. They may also be able to help you clarify your sound needs. (For exact help, look under "Sound Systems and Equipment—Renting.")

If your budget is too small to rent at all, then contact area schools, churches, and colleges to arrange a plan to borrow their equipment in exchange for free advertisement in your bulletin/programs. These people are usually very cooperative to churches if they're assured that responsible care will be given to their equipment. Before contacting these lighting designers, familiarize yourself with the types of lighting equipment mentioned in the coming paragraph, or see the glossary at the end of this book. Be prepared to discuss such equipment as Lekos (Ellipsodial), Fresnels, Pars, Dimmers, Lowel Omnis and Totas, Scoops, Strips or Bars, Cyc Lights, and Follow Spots. Remember too to ask about colored gels and cinefoil.

To help you discover the typical lighting needs for a production, let's study *The Healing*, which called for various types of lights. It was a much more challenging play to light than to amplify with sound, due mainly to the fade-ins and fade-outs of each flashback scene. Also the script calls for various mood changes that colored lighting helps to bring about. Since the play was staged in a gymnasium, our lights were pre-set days before the play opened. Therefore, adding colored gels to the existing stagelights for a sudden mood change was impossible *during* a performance.

Instead, normal stage lights, plus a separate set of lights with colored gels, were hung and with the use of a dimmer board, normal stage lights were dimmed, and the deep-colored gel lights were raised during special scenes. This use of a dimmer board is very effective in lighting mood changes and in fading to a blackout at the end of certain scenes. Par Lights were mainly used to light *The Healing*. Pars are round lights, approximately two feet long that have built-in reflectors in the bulb and come in sizes of 48, 56, and 64.

If your facility does not have built in stage-lighting, Par lights are efficient and uncomplicated pieces of equipment. When lighting a stage it is always best to project light onto the front of the actors (for visibility), but also to illuminate them from behind (to help eliminate shadows and also to help distinguish the actors from their backgrounds). Colored gels are easily used in Pars, and in "normal" stage lighting, a light shade of pink enhances actors' complexions and gives them a healthy glow. (Rosco's "no-color-pink" is what we used.) A blue-tinted gel (Rosco's "full-blue") is also helpful in softening the harsh glare of a spotlight and can be used for the majority of the play's action.

The rocking-chair scene that ends Act I of *The Healing* was lit with another type of light. Using two Lekos (an Ellipsodial projector in which the exact direction of its light can easily be pinpointed), one was used to light the front of the chair and another illuminated it from behind, using deep-pink, colored gels to enhance Claudia's reflective monologue. A dimmer board gradually replaced the normal stage lighting to this deep pink shade, and the scene was intensified greatly. Two Lowel Omni lights were used on the auxiliary, or flashback, stage since the scrim's lighting had to be so carefully controlled. When the scrim (see glossary) was lit from the front, it remained an obscure barrier to the audience, and the stage behind it was invisible. When a flashback scene occurred, the dimmer was used to remove the front lighting and to bring up the four Fresnels (LTM Pepper 650's, two for front light and two for back lighting), which hung behind the scrim and lit the auxiliary stage. This change of lighting made the scrim transparent, and the flashback stage could magically appear at any desired moment. (Sky cyes are also effective on backwashing scrims.)

During Act II, Scene 3, when Ethan discovers Annie's illness, we chose to create a chilling mood by having snow fall outside the family living-room window. (Stage snow can be purchased at any stagecraft shop.) A piece of material was hung in the window's background, and then a potted tree was placed to one side for added dimension. When the snow was released slowly from above the window, two lights were used to make sure the snow was visible to such a large audience. Lighting the snow from above was a Lowel Tota with a blue gel for accent. Lighting the snow from the ground up, a Lowel Omni was used with a white gel for clarity. Just as back and front lights assure crisp visibility of an actor, top and bottom lights assure the visibility of your tiny snowflakes. Another consideration for your lighting needs are your "houselights," or the lighting provided to illuminate the gym with a soft dinner mood. Four Lowel Tota lights were hung on the gym ceiling's four main beams. Aiming straight up toward the ceiling, the light bounced back down to the audience for a very soothing eating atmosphere. This reflection-lighting style also eliminated most of the heat the audience would have had to bear with direct light. (Again, a dimmer was used to bring houselights up and down for the beginnings and endings of each Act.)

A final consideration when hanging your lights, especially in a large auditorium with a raised stage, is to regard your audience when you light your stage. Remember they are looking up and onto the stage and that you must somehow aim your glaring lights downward without shining them into your audience members' eyes. This can most easily be accomplished by hanging the lights as high as possible and at the steepest angle possible. This way you are sure to light only the stage and not your audience. Still, if your audience is being flooded by lights and your equipment has no barndoors (the adjustable flaps on the sides of your light that curb the amount and shape of light projected from the front of your spotlight), then create your own barndoors by purchasing a product called Cinefoil. It is a black, heavy, shapeable foil which, when placed on the front area of your spotlight, allows you to control exactly where you want light to be cast.

In review, *The Healing* required nine Pars, three for front-stage light using the "full-blue" gel; three for backstage light, using the "full-blue" gel; three Pars for front-stage lighting, using "no-color-pink" gels to enhance complexions and makeup), two Lekos, or Ellipsodials (for front and back illumination of the rocking-chair scene, both with deep-pink gels), four Lowel Tota lights for houselights, one Lowel Tota with blue gel for the snow, one Lowel Omni with white gel for the snow, four Fresnels for the scrim/auxiliary stage area (all four were LTM Pepper 650's with pink gels, two for front lights and two for back lights), and two Lowel Omni's which lit the front of the scrim, keeping it cloudy until desired otherwise.

Additional Technical Needs: Although only three or four men were actually running lights and sound during each performance of *The Healing*, many more men volunteered their time for hanging lights and for securing microphones. Following is a breakdown of each technical and production crew needed to produce *The Healing* in the First Baptist Church of Donelson's Family life Center. Keep in mind that if your group and performance area are smaller, you may not need as much lighting and amplification, thus reducing your need for so many technicians.

"Confess your trespasses to one another, and pray for one another, that you may be healed" James 5:16

THE HEALING by Laura Harris Smith

OUR CAST (in order of appearance)

Tommy Long	as	Emmett Lee Westbrook
Madeline S. White	as	Dorothy Oakes
Donna Merritt	as	Grace Ann Westbrook
Dan Borsos	as	Young Emmett Westbrook
Ashley Crook	as	Young Millicent
Tyler McCulloch	as	Young Ethan
Courtney Crook	as	Young Annie
Drew Ann Borsos	as	Millicent Kae Adams
Paul McCulloch	as	Ethan Murray Westbrook
Laura H. Smith	as	Charlotte Ann Scott
Stephanie M. Harmon	as	Claudia Carney
Jessica Smith	as	Emma Lee Scott
Rachel Harmon	as	Young Claudia
Megan McCulloch	as	Young Grace Murray
Don Joines	as	Dr. Martin Grayson

The carolers - Sherrie Allen, Randy Barron, Jill Fry, Steve Hall, Teresa Houser, Bill Malone.

The mainstage setting for THE HEALING is the Westbrook home in Brookport, Illinois, resting just on the Illinois / Kentucky border, population 1,128.

Act I - Friday, December 22, 1989
Act II - Scenes 1-5, Sunday, Christmas Eve
Scene 6 - Christmas morning 1989

TECHNICAL AND PRODUCTION CREWS

Director and producer————————————————Laura Harris Smith
Co-Director Special Scenes————————————————Beth Ryan
Stage Manager————————————————Julie Hearne
Properties Manager————————————————Theresa Rasmussen
Lighting Foreman————————————————David Roche
Sound foreman————————————————Mike Hearne
Technical Support Specialist————————————————Ken Porter
Technical Crew————————————David Fry, Al Green, Paul Nichols,
Robert Lunn, Jimmy Startup,
Allen Tack, Mark Campbell,
Mike Carey, and Ron Gasser
Set Design————————————————Laura H. Smith
Julie Hearne
Set Crew————————————————Jill Fry,
David Fry
Phyllis Dye
Kerry Dye
Set Construction Foreman————————————————David Fry
Mike Hearne
Chris Smith
Makeup / Image Consultant————————————————Sondra Turner
Children's Backstage Assistance————————————————Donna Merritt
House Managers————————————————Carole McCulloch
Paula McCulloch
Ushers————————————————Bryan Thornhill
Heather Laxton
Stephen Fisher
Kitchen Managers————————————————Julia Forester
Pat Berkley
Carla Green
Donna Winfree
"THE HEALING" Logo Design————————————————Tim Smith
Publicity Coordinators————————————————Beth Ryan
Laura H. Smith
Drew Ann Borsos
Reservationists————————————Drew Ann Borsos, Stephanie Harmon,
Don Joines, Laura H. Smith,
and Madeline White
Program Flyer and Printing————————————————Karen Waddell
Video Editor————————————————Steve Rasmussen

Other crew jobs not listed here include organizing the catered meal, scheduling the photographer for publicity shots, hiring a florist for all stage floral arrangements, and dinner theatre house-table centerpieces, plus co-ordinating all set and furniture donations. These simple responsibilities need not require a separate committee each. Instead the director/producer can easily coordinate these affairs unless he or she desires assistance. A costume designer may also be required for your production but was not essential for this play.

Notice also that this play required a co-director for special scenes. This probably won't be necessary for your group, unless your director also decides to become a part of the cast, as was the case in our show this one year! Whenever a director is absent from directing and instead on the stage acting, a co-director should be considered in order to preserve good direction for those scenes.

In Chapter 5, The Director's Chair, a detailed job description is laid out for the director. However, using the previous technical- and production-crew list from *The Healing*, let's also study each committee and discover exactly what is expected from each of these.

Stage Manager. Next to the director this person has sole responsibility for all the actors and helps them to enter on time for all stage cues. During the actual performances, he or she serves in a director's capacity back-stage, since the director is most likely to be seated in the audience.

Properties Manager (Props). This party locates and manages any hand-held items the actors may require during their performances. These items are referred to as "props," and the props manager must not only locate or make them, but must also organize them onto the prop table. This table houses all carry-on objects and is located just behind the stage entrance for easy access by the actors. Along with helping the actors quickly find their props, the prop manager may have also aided the director in locating various smaller stage decorations.

Lighting Foreman. This person should be technically skilled in lighting of some kind. He should be familiar with how to determine your lighting needs, how to find or rent the needed equipment, and most importantly, how to operate it. Since this is your greatest area of technical need, this person must be responsible, as well as able to work well with the many people he will have to staff.

Sound Foreman. Just like the lighting foreman, your sound man needs to be accustomed to and aware of the latest in sound technology. He will be able to assist you with all your amplification needs, as well as coordinate all offstage cues (phone rings, doorbells, special effects, musical cues, etc.).

Technical-support Specialist. This is usually one person who offers his or her expertise in a certain technical field. In a sense, this person may serve as an assistant to the lighting or sound foremen.

Technical Crew. These individuals are helpful to the lighting and sound foremen in the hanging of the lights and the placement of microphones. In addition, some of them may need to be present during the actual perform-ances to offer assistance.

Set Designer. This person, sometimes the director, carefully studies the script and determines how to best design the stage and decorate it.

Set Crew. This crew, along with the director, is responsible for finding the set's furniture. During the performances this crew also makes any set changes that are necessary.

Set Construction Foremen. Occasionally, pieces of the stage must be built or added onto. Men specializing in elbow grease (and carpentry!) can help meet any set construction needs the production has.

Makeup/Hair. For the final dress rehearsal and the performances, the actors will need to be in full stage makeup that is applied by a skilled makeup technician. He or she should be somewhat familiar with the process of aging a character with makeup. In general, however, this technician will simply assist the actors in coordinating their individual makeup needs. Also, their appearances need to be double-checked to be sure that the harsh stage lights do not cause any of the actors to appear "washed-out" when they are on stage.

Children's Backstage Assistance. If children make up a large part of your cast, then they will not need to be left unattended backstage. A backstage mother will not only help keep them occupied, but will also help them remember their cues and entrances.

House Manager. Your theatre performance space, or "house," will need to be under one person's close supervision during performances. This manager should be friendly and diplomatic, as he or she will stand at the door and greet each guest, taking his or his ticket. Next, the house manager assigns an usher to take each visitor to his or her seat. But, in the event that two people claim the same seat, the House Manager must be able to tactfully discern who first purchased the seat, and then try to find an alternate table for the other guest. In such a case, you can see where it would be beneficial to have two house managers so the entrance is never left unattended.

Ushers. These people see each dinner-theatre guest to his or her seat and provide them with a program for their ease in viewing and becoming familiar with the play. This is often an area where teenagers enjoy serving, and they need only be responsible and courteous.

Kitchen Managers. Working closely with the caterer, these individuals remain in the kitchen before the performances and help dish all the food onto the plates. As they prepare the plates, the cast takes them via trays and serves the food to their assigned audience tables in character.

Logo Designer. Finding a person who is skilled in computer graphics will be of great service to you in the creative design of your programs, flyers, and tickets.

Publicity Coordinator. Hanging flyers, contacting local radio and television stations for free advertisement, mailing flyers to churches, schools, and colleges, etc. These are just a few of the ways that a publicity coordinator can effectively advertise your dinner theatre for next to nothing.

Reservationists. These are the contact people for purchasing tickets while they are on sale. In the church setting, they mainly wait immediately outside the sanctuary before and after each service so the church members have easy access to tickets. This process usually requires at least two people, since each time a ticket is sold the customer must view a seating chart, choose a seat, pay for his ticket, then have his table and seat number recorded on both a master guest list and his individual ticket. If childcare is being provided by your church, he must also give you information on each child and pay for the childcare at this same time. Since long lines are quite possible, having plenty of reservationists is wise. (One of these reservationists should also be one of your church office workers since he or she will need to be familiar with ticket sales when customers stop by the church office to purchase tickets.)

Program and Flyer Printing. Once your logo designer helps you create your programs, flyers, and tickets, this individual purchases your desired colored paper and prints these materials for you.

Video Editor. Usually part of the technical crew, this person captures the play's performance on video tape to be placed in your church library for ministering purposes. Those families who were unable to attend the play can view it simply by checking out the video, but you'll be surprised by how many of these families are second- and third-time viewers!

If in any of your productions you see the need for a committee or crew not described in this chapter, then by all means create one! There's no limit to the amount of technical and production crews you may have as long as they are all well-managed and understand that they must communicate closely with and report financially to the director.

Thank these crews often for their hard work. Remind your cast to work patiently with them as they labor to technically accent each moment of your play. And finally, remember that these precious people get no curtain call, but they deserve a standing ovation. Make sure that they get one from you.

(Special thanks is given to David Roche for his collaboration on this chapter.)

8

Creating the Dinner Theatre Mood:

A Memorable Experience for All the Senses!

Long before the curtain rises on your play, your guests should already have exercised each of their five senses and applied them toward the dinner-theatre experience.

Imagine that you are a guest at your own dinner theatre. You are greeted at the door by the *touch* of a welcome hand that not only takes your ticket, but shakes your hand and thanks you for your patronage. As an usher escorts you into the "house" and to your seat, you are invited to relax and unwind to the *sound* of soothing music. As you wait, mixing and fellowshiping with the others at your table, the luring aroma of simmering food captures your attention and rouses your appetite.

Suddenly, the *smell* draws nearer, as does the *sight* of a face that looks very familiar. "Hey, could that be Max? You know, the Max that's in our class. I think he's headed over here with our food. It is! It is Max! I didn't know he was in this play. Hi, Max!" Slowly, Max looks over his shoulder as if confused, and then responds calmly, "I'm sorry, Sir, you must have mistaken me for someone else. My name is Emmett Lee Westbrook, and I will be your waiter tonight. Please enjoy your meal and if there's anything I can get you, don't hesitate to ask." You are pleasantly dumbfounded. You were sure that was Max. Of course, he must've started wearing makeup and strange clothes, but still, that had to be him. Thank goodness someone at your table turns through the program and confirms it. "The part of Emmett Lee Westbrook will be played by Maxwell Cooper." As you all laugh, you focus once again on the savory spread that's just been served. One *taste* confirms it: You're already glad you came.

Without having even seen the play, your guests will have a "sixth sense" that they are going to love it. This chapter will temporarily disregard your actual presentation and concern itself with every detail that precedes it.

After selecting your dinner-theatre play, read it repeatedly for underlying themes and dominant moods. Then consider the following elements of your dinner theatre and apply those themes and moods toward them. (Examples are cited from performances of *The Inçentive* and *The Healing.*)

(1) Logo Design for Advertisement Flyers. To ensure that you have an audience, really jazz up your flyers to entice people to take notice of them. An interesting flyer equals an interesting play to the viewer, so start with a catchy logo. This logo should serve as a quick commercial for your play and its underlying themes and dominant moods.

THE HEALING *THE HEALING*

"Confess your trespasses to one another, and pray for one another, that you may be healed." James 5:16

Shown here is the logo created for *The Healing*, followed by an enticing description, or blurb, about the play's storyline. The full flyer is found in Chapter 11, Budgeting and Publicity, but for right now, let's study why this logo was chosen. The larger lettering which spells "The Healing" appears first with a very faint "T," and the letters gradually restore their intended color along the way, ending with a bold, solid "G." Concealed with "The Healing" is a smaller "the healing," using the darkest, most confident lettering yet. All of this is symbolic, of course, of the restoration process that occurs within the boundaries of all physical, emotional, and spiritual healings.

This design was created by computer using simple logo graphics software. Any graphic artist can work with you to render such a representative logo, but you really need not spend the money to hire a professional. With the purchase of simple graphic software, most churches have the computer hardware to generate many high-quality logo-design alternatives for your play. This keeps costs minimal, especially if you are computer friendly and can serve as your own graphic artist. If you're not so brave, or are just limited in time, allow a computer friend to take creative control of the logo design after you've communicated to him the play's themes and moods. If computers are altogether out of the question for your tiny group, then simply forfeit the computer graphics and find yourself a reliable artist. Your logo need not be fancy for it to be symbolic.

(2) Color choices for programs and flyers. The exact logo you used on your flyers should also be showcased on your programs or bulletins. Likewise, you should choose a uniform color for both, to enable your audience to quickly identify them with your play. Is there a recurring color that is mentioned throughout the play? Does the play's title cite a particular color or bring one to mind? Ask these questions before selecting your flyer and program color. Throughout *The Incentive* a relentless pursuit for a lavender piano was always on the mind of the pompous Kelly Ann Acklen. Therefore, the color lavender was an undeniable choice for flyer and program color.

(3) Ushers' attire. Suggest to your ushers that they dress according to the time period of your play. Does your play take place in nineteenth century New England? Then find long skirts for the women ushers and knickers for the men! Perhaps your play is present day, but is set in the Deep South. In that cast, have your ushers polish a Southern drawl and pour it on thick!

(4) Music. Of course, your play should include music that's appropriate for its individual scenes and the curtain call. But don't forget the mood-setting dinner music! Set the scene for what your guests will see by providing for them music that has a similar mood or that is from the same time period your play is set in.

(5) Table Centerpieces. All the tables in your dinner theatre should be decorated with matching centerpieces. These centerpieces are not mere table decorations, but instead are your audience's first clue about your play's content. Skim through your play for important symbolism or for tangible articles of significance. At the end of *The Healing*, Emmett Westbrook's character finally makes a much-needed transformation, compelling him to send Dory, age fifty-six, her very first bouquet of roses. This tangible symbol of Emmett's healing was expressed best by placing a single red rose in a vase on each dinner theatre table. When Dory received her roses on stage, the audience members were able to experience the same beauty and fragrance of that magical moment right at their own tables.

(6) Time and season changes in the play. Unless your play's story takes place over a few days, your audience may experience temporary confu-

sion during the progression of your play's scenes. This may be especially true if your play spans several months or years. Of course, with close attention, they'll eventually catch on, but there is no reason why you cannot creatively assist them. Creative assistance in understanding time progression does not include in-between-scene walk-ins carrying date and time cue cards!

Instead, take advantage of your dinner theatre tables and change the centerpieces during intermission to indicate a time or season change. For instance, *The Inȼentive* spans a full year and has three season changes. Act I begins at Thanksgiving, and our centerpieces reflected a harvest theme. Act II, however, takes place four months later—in the spring. So during intermission the harvest baskets were replaced with baskets of fresh, fragrant potpourri. Then, Scene 5 jumps ahead seven months without much dialogue to indicate that autumn has returned. So, table-runners were assigned to visit each table during the blackout before Scene 5 and sprinkle each table with dried autumn leaves that we had purchased from a stagecraft shop. The audience immediately understood that fall had returned and this was important to the play's plot. They were so eager for the beginning of Scene 5 you could have heard a pin drop!

(7) Plate and flatware coordination. Your facility may have access to enough place settings (including plates, cups, and silverware) to accommodate your guests. If you have this luxury, then by all means use it in this age of ecology awareness. (Reusable, washable plates and utensils will also save your dinner theatre hundreds of dollars!) If this is your plan, you can still coordinate your table colors by purchasing reusable, colored-plastic or cloth tablecloths available at your area party store.

If disposable plates are the route you choose, your table will be more colorful, but be sure to allow a large part of your budget for this expense. Find durable, colorful plates that can withstand being handled by the caterer, the kitchen managers, your cast/waiters, and finally, your guests. Think of the plate and napkin colors as an extension of the colors you've selected to represent your play through the printed flyers and programs. Of course, sometimes this color may not be available in or appropriate for table decorations. In that case, coordinate your plates, napkins, and table-cloths with your centerpieces. In *The Healing* durable rose-wine plates topped a sleek, white-plastic tablecloth and were accented with a rose and baby's breath centerpiece.

(8) Actors serve the meal in character. As described at the beginning of the chapter, audience members are delighted when they're given opportu-

nity to interact with the cast. Of course, they are stunned when served by a good friend who denies knowing them. Still, this format gives the audience a quick overview of the cast and makes them eager for the play to begin. As a suggestion, count the tables in your dinner theatre and divide them equally among your cast members. If there are a few tables left over, give the more responsible and speedy actors an extra table each. Even the children in your play can serve a table, especially if you assign them a table with a short walking distance from the kitchen. As an extra surprise for your dinner theatre guests, search through your players for any characters with professional occupations (i.e., lawyers, doctors, etc.). Then, using plain-white, heavy-stock paper, type and cut out personalized business cards for your characters to distribute to the guests they serve and to whom they introduce themselves. The audiences of *The In¢entive* appreciated these mementos given to them by Lillian Laraby, attorney at law, by Lesley Kelly, owner of Kelly's Piano Parlour, and by Wilson Foster, pastor of Gibsonville First Baptist Church.

(9) Your meal. This worthwhile subject, since it is half of the dinner theatre experience, deserves an entire chapter's attention. Chapter 9 is devoted to just that and should be read carefully. However, it is worth mentioning here that this, too, is one of the areas you must heedfully plan only after searching your play for any and all clues. Does anyone in your play eat on stage, and if so, does the script mention what they're eating? If so, then surprise your audience by serving them the same menu, as was done in *The Incentive* when the viewers joined the cast in a full Thanksgiving meal. (This was also successful in *The Healing* when the audience was served all of Emmett Westbrook's favorite foods as prepared by Dory at the tense family reunion.) If the script does not mention food, then consider the location of your play. A full Cajun meal would highlight any Louisiana-based play just as Italian cuisine would perfectly suit a play set in Rome. A third option is to consider any ethnic backgrounds emphasized in your play. If your play's main characters are Japanese, then by all means break out the chopsticks!

(10) Information Tables. To underscore major issues dealt with during your play, provide for your guests a helpful information table which offers community and ministry assistance to these needs. If your dinner theatre plans to produce *The Healing* then consider supplying an information table with informative brochures on Huntington's Disease, supplied free by the Huntington's Disease Society of America (listed under 1-800 Directory Assistance). Single parenting, divorce, and the dysfunctional family are all

crucial topics in the play, so your information table should be stocked with counseling and ministering material which promotes your community- and family-support groups. Finally, be prepared to distribute to your interested viewers, practical information on the hearing impaired and perhaps even copies of the American Sign Language Alphabet. This would not only educate them in a valuable form of communication, but it would also afford your deaf guests with instant fellowship. Also, if you anticipate a large crowd of hearing-impaired visitors, then try to seat them together and provide them with a signer/interpreter.

When all is said and done, make sure that your entire dinner-theatre environment has fit your play as snugly as a glove. Year after year, the guests who visit your dinner theatre will leave not only feeling entertained and perhaps ministered to, but they'll also sense a true professionalism about your well-planned production. Your audiences will come to expect it, and you can be sure they will notice and even inform you of any details you've overlooked!

9

The Dinner

Half of a Good Dinner Theatre
Is Its Dinner!

With the dozens of hours your cast will spend rehearsing the play you've selected, you owe it to yourselves to be absolutely sure the meal you serve will be equally as polished. If you enjoy entertaining guests, then just think of the dinner theatre house as your home, and imagine you are inviting hundreds of guests over for a full dinner! Each guest deserves special attention and a warm meal, and that's exactly what they'll receive if you plan the menu carefully.

Your Menu: With the help of this chapter, you'll be able to decide if a caterer or a covered-dish dinner theatre is best for your group. But regardless of how your food is supplied, you will still have to first plan a menu that suits your play, your audience's needs, and your budget. As discussed in Chapter 8, search your play for setting, ethnic background of characters, or any foods mentioned in the script. These helpful hints can provide you with some creative ideas on tying your menu into your play. Maybe none of the above are mentioned in the play you've selected, but you know the play takes place during the Thanksgiving season, as in *The Incentive.* In that case, include your guests in the celebration by serving them a fall Thanksgiving meal.

As a guide, try to offer your guests a meat, or meat dish, two vegetables, bread, an iced beverage (tea), and a dessert. This is a standard request when working with a caterer. If you are finding it difficult to hire a caterer whose charge per plate is lower than your ticket price, then negotiate on the drink or the dessert, and ask for volunteers to supply these for your dinner theatre. However, don't do this too quickly, because there is no reason why an affordable caterer cannot be found. If necessary, search for a reliable yet new caterer to your area. Chances are he would be more interested in publicity instead of profit.

Caterers: If your dinner theatre is serving a crowd of 100 or more guests, you need to consider hiring a caterer. Although you will creatively decide what your meal should include, your caterer will be able to offer practical suggestions to aid you in your final menu selections. For example, from experience he may know that keeping pasta hot for 500 guests is next to impossible, so listen to his advice. The smaller your cast and kitchen area is, the slower your guests will be served. So try to serve foods that retain their heat for several minutes, and be prepared to courteously reheat an occasional plate for a dissatisfied guest.

Most caterers prefer to cook all the food they will serve at their own private locations, transporting it to your dinner theatre just prior to your production. The food is kept hot in their numerous aluminum storage containers and then dished onto the plates immediately before the audience is served. Caterers provide many other services besides the meal, such as staffing workers to help dish the food onto the plates. They also are accustomed to serving the food they've prepared. Thus, when you inform your caterer that you'll be staffing your own volunteer kitchen managers to dish food and that they will hand the plates directly to the cast members who will serve the meal, then his charge per plate is sure to decrease. Remember to discuss any necessary condiments with your caterer, such as salt, pepper, sauces, salad dressings, sugar and alternative sweeteners, and margarine or butter. Also, if your facility doesn't have an industrial ice machine then inform your caterer he must supply the ice. These details seem very tedious, especially if you dwell on the fact that you'll be serving hundreds of people and trying to please each of them. Remember that no one person can handle that alone, and that through the delegation of work to your caterer, the kitchen managers, and the cast, each of your dinner guests will receive the individual attention they deserve.

Covered-Dish Dinner Theatre Perhaps you are planning a smaller production due to a limited performance and seating area in your facility. Of course, the smaller your production, the fewer your expenses will be. But if you still don't expect to break even after paying your caterer, then consider a covered-dish donation dinner theatre. To help project if your dinner-theatre production will break even or make money, apply this formula:

1. **TICKET PRICE MINUS CATERER PER PLATE PRICE = PROFIT PER PERSON.**
2. **PROFIT PER PERSON X AUDITORIUM CAPACITY X NUMBER OF PERFORMANCES PLANNED = TOTAL DINNER THEATRE PROFIT.**

(For more helpful budgeting information, refer to Chapter 11, Publicity and Budgeting.)

If this total figure is insufficient in covering your play's total expenses, you have two options. Either raise your ticket price or lower your play's expenses. Raise your ticket price as a last resort. Your play's expenses can be cut in one of two areas: (1) the dinner: find a cheaper way to provide the meal, or (2) the theatre: a cheaper production; spend less on costumes props, set, etc.

Also, scheduling more performances will increase your profit. As expected, the preferred route is to try first to cut your costs, and this is easily done by reducing the largest expense you'll have: the meal. If you cannot match a caterer to your budget, or if you prefer to bypass that course altogether, then appoint a covered-dish coordinator to organize the meal. Ticket price, of course, should decrease by probably half, with the added entry fee of a covered dish.

Once the tickets have been sold and your guests can be counted, the covered-dish coordinator contacts every ticket buyer and arranges for each to bring a certain dish. Naturally, this method works best with smaller crowds. Also, keeping the menu consistent is important so each audience member will have the same foods. Kitchen managers will organize foods according to matching groups, and then dish the food onto the plates just as they would if the caterer had brought the prepared food. Remember that even though your ticket price has been greatly reduced, all monies acquired from a covered-dish dinner theatre are pure profit! In addition, your profits stand a great chance of being doubled!

Kitchen Managers. By now you know that these individuals are vital to the success of your dinner. In the church setting, volunteers who are familiar with your facility's kitchen are best-qualified for this job. Because your caterer will not be familiar with your kitchen's design, the kitchen managers will be very helpful in assisting him with locating special items and utilizing and maximizing all work spaces. Since the director will be unable to be present in the kitchen on performance nights, the kitchen managers become directors of the dining experience, serving as mediators between the caterer, who prepares the food, and the cast, who serves it. They will also have the primary responsibility of transferring the caterer's food to plates and of filling glasses with ice and the drink you have chosen. (Iced tea is a good crowd-pleaser; however, always have pitchers of ice-water on hand.) As the plates and cups are being filled, the actors return to the kitchen with their trays and then serve them to the audience members at the table they've been assigned. Kitchen managers also have cleanup responsibility, though, with the use of disposable plates and cups, cleanup is always minimal. Remember the weight of the kitchen manager's job when you are selecting these individuals, but also remember to acknowledge their value to your production at each and every performance.

Cast Members Serve In Character. Remember Max from Chapter 8? In section eight of that chapter, the dinner theatre tradition of actors' serving the meal in character was discussed. Never underestimate the part this plays in your complete dinner theatre production. Your audience has come expecting to be fed and entertained, but they are pleasantly rattled when they realize they are face to face with a member of your cast! What's more, that actor may be a familiar friend or even a family member to that audience guest, but is not allowed to break character and speak to the audience member as an acquaintance. If the character one actress portrays is a cranky, malicious gossip, then she should serve her table in an accommodating matter but without an overly-friendly attitude. Caution should be used, however, since the guests do need to feel welcome. The safest compromise is for this cranky, malicious gossip to serve her guests while gossiping about a fellow character who is serving a nearby table. In addition, never reveal the play's ending by having a cast member serve in the character mood they will transform into by the play's end. In other words, even if the cranky, malicious gossip changes her ways during the play, she should serve the meal as she is first portrayed. The serving of the meal also benefits the actors in overcoming any stage fright they may be experiencing at the beginning of each performance. Allowing them to interact with their audience takes the edge off of that adrenalin rush all actors experience, and it also ignites an enthusiasm with the crowd for the performance to begin.

The director is responsible for assigning dinner theatre tables to each actor, trying first to divide them equally. If your dinner theatre accommodates thirty-five tables, but you have only seventeen actors in the play, then assign each actor two tables, leaving one extra. Choose one swift, responsible actor and assign him three tables, saving him some leg work by placing him closest to the kitchen. Child actors make excellent waiters also.

However, they, too, should be placed next to the kitchen to prevent major spills. Sometimes, special health conditions of a particular character will determine which tables he or she is assigned. For instance, if a wheelchair is part of one character's performance, then allow the actor to serve his tables in the chair, using another character's assistance if necessary and staying as close to the kitchen as possible.

In the long run, anyone could argue that easier serving methods could be found. A self-serving buffet is one no-maintenance route to feeding large crowds. However, not only does regulating crowd portions and repeated helpings pose a difficult challenge, but the buffet format cheats the audience and the cast of the intimate interaction they both need.

In closing, envision the five areas mentioned here before finalizing any plans for your dinner. The menu you choose should complement both your audience and your play. The caterer or covered-dish coordinator you appoint to develop that menu should be qualified and adaptable. Kitchen managers handling the food should be organized and efficient since they'll be working within a time limit. In addition, the cast, or waiters, will require equal diligence, as well as patience, as they culminate the entire process. Whatever your specific needs, and whatever method you choose to realize your menu, make certain they do justice to your entire dinner theatre production. Don't forget that half of a good dinner theatre is *dinner!*

10

Acting

By the time your dinner theatre has been scheduled, the play you've selected has been cast, the menu has been coordinated, and the set is being built, the director may feel more like a coordinator than a creative drama director. Despite the organization the production must have, it must not lack in creative soundness.

Primarily, the actors have the task of realizing the play's full potential through their character study and scene development. However, if each actor on stage in a particular scene has a different interpretation of that scene's mood, then the director must quickly intervene with guidance in the proper direction. This will happen less often if the actors have been well-educated in the areas of character motivation and in discovering scene objectives. Since most actors in the church arena are amateurs, the director will be responsible for training them in these areas. Once the cast has been formed, perhaps an entire rehearsal should be devoted to discussing acting technique. It will save rehearsal time in the long run, and the actors will enjoy the opportunity of making their own discoveries. So where is the starting point for Acting 101? Unfortunately (or fortunately) there is no formula for acting, since it is an emotional experience—but there are certain disciplines that, when followed, can cause creativity to abound quickly.

After the play has been blocked and actual rehearsing rehearsals have begun, introducing creative acting methods will be well-received by the actors. In fact, by now they should be eager to fully understand their characters.

First, distribute copies of the following questions, Discovering Your Character's Objectives. Give your actors one week to complete the questions and return them. This will propel the actors quicker than anything as they will finally be thinking and searching independently for their characters' significances to the plot.

DISCOVERING YOUR CHARACTER'S OBJECTIVES

CHARACTER HISTORY

1. WHAT IS YOUR CHARACTER'S NAME?
2. HOW OLD ARE YOU?
3. WHAT DO YOU DO IN LIFE? OCCUPATION?
4. ARE YOU ACHIEVING WHAT YOU WANT OUT OF LIFE?
5. WHAT WAS YOUR EARLY FAMILY LIFE LIKE? (SIZE, YOUR BIRTH ORDER, ETC.)
6. WHAT ARE YOUR PERSONAL OPINIONS OR BELIEFS?
7. WHAT DO YOU ENJOY THE MOST? THE LEAST?
8. ARE YOU AN HONEST PERSON? DO YOU USUALLY SAY WHAT YOU MEAN?
9. HOW DO OTHER CHARACTERS TREAT YOU? WHY?
10. STATE YOUR INVOLVEMENT WITH ALL OTHER CHARACTERS.
11. NAME CERTAIN ACTIONS IN THE PLAY THAT DEFINE YOUR CHARACTER.
12. WHAT TRANSFORMATIONS DOES YOUR CHARACTER MAKE IN THE PLAY?

MOTIVATIONAL QUESTIONS

(TO BE ANSWERED CLEARLY FOR ALL OF THE SCENES IN WHICH YOU ARE IN)

1. WHY AM I HERE?
2. DO I NEED SOMETHING OR DOES SOMEONE NEED ME?
3. WHAT IS MY RELATIONSHIP TO EACH PERSON HERE?
4. HOW DID I GET HERE?
5. WHERE WAS I BEFORE I CAME HERE? WHY?
6. WHY DID I LEAVE THERE?
7. AM I COMFORTABLE WHERE I AM NOW?

SPIRITUAL QUESTIONS

(ANSWER BEFORE EACH PERFORMANCE—THEN FOLLOW WITH A CHARACTER QUIET TIME, DEVOTION, AND THEN PRAYER.)

1. IS YOUR CHARACTER A CHRISTIAN? FOR HOW LONG? ARE YOU BACKSLIDDEN OR GROWING?
2. ARE YOU CONTRIBUTING TO THE CONFLICT OF THE PLAY OF ARE YOU A VICTIM OF SPIRITUAL WARFARE?
3. HOW COULD GOD BE TRYING TO USE YOUR CHARACTER IN HIS OR HER SETTING?
4. YOUR CHARACTER'S ACTIONS, AND CONSEQUENCES OF HIS OR HER ACTIONS, WILL SERVE AS AN INFLUENCE TO YOUR AUDIENCE. FIRST, WILL THIS INFLUENCE BE GOOD OR BAD? AND SECOND, WHAT LESSON WILL THEY LEARN FROM YOU?

Before the worksheets are returned, begin scheduling an individual private meeting with each cast member. In these meetings (before or after rehearsal time) discuss in detail any character questions the actor may have, plus any personal needs they may have, including prayer requests. An actor is more likely to confide in the director and ask detailed questions when meeting privately.

During the course of completing the worksheets and individual cast-member meetings, set aside one rehearsal, or part of one, for a crash course in rehearsing techniques. Require everyone's attendance and yet keep the meeting's topic a secret. Bring some refreshments and ask that everyone get comfortable on the floor or in a circle of chairs as you provide for them the following techniques. Stress to them the significance of applying and utilizing these techniques and even furnish them with materials necessary to take adequate notes. This rehearsal will be a welcome break for the actors, especially as they are selected to participate in the impromptu exercises listed ahead.

Primarily, the quickest route from inexperienced acting to experienced acting is learning *how* to experience, period. Of course, as living beings we each have the ability to think, feel, and react with emotion, so this craft does not have to be learned but rather tapped into when performing.

Konstantin Stanislavski (born K. Sergeyevich Alexeyev) was a Russian director and actor who authored numerous books and biographies, including *An Actor's Handbook, Building a Character*, and *Stanislavski in Rehearsal*. Stanislavski's famous "Method Acting" technique trained actors to enhance their performances by studying the inner lives of their characters as if they were real people. Naturally, by living the life of a character on stage, the actor loses the tendency towards a rigid, hollow portrayal and the mere recital of lines.

Building from Stanislavski's "Method Acting," the Christian actor can find even deeper motivation, such as spiritual objectives for his or her character. With your cast assembled, present the following facts before discussing any actual techniques.

A. As a cast, we are not professional, real-live actors. Unfortunately, our audience will be professional real-live people expecting us to do more than recite our lines and walk to our designated spots. They'll quickly discern if our emotions are insincere, or worse, missing.

B. (Call for a volunteer.) Recall a play you once saw. Now try to imagine the exact costumes used and every lighting technique in detail. This cannot be done!

C. Now name what can be recalled about the same play mentioned. Generally a play's theme is easily remembered. Also, audience members will look back on a certain character and how they changed from the play's start to its finish. They remember their own emotional journeys as they related to these certain characters.

D. Therefore, the actor must be convincing in his role. Some people are under the misconception that the director designs the set, costumes, lights, and sound to impress the audience. On the contrary, these elements are used for their effect on the actors. That effect should be to enhance each actor's concentration while on stage.

Once the actors and actresses in your dinner theatre understand that they are responsible for communicating with their audience and not serving as a flashy spectacle to them, they'll desire to know how to stay tuned into the audience. The following ideas are essential:

1. Concentration on Stage. As if this task weren't hard enough, the actor on stage may not get the adequate help he needs from his fellow actors who are watching him rehearse. How can they help? Their silence is priceless to him. After his rehearsal, he then needs to hear feedback from them, something they cannot offer if they haven't given him their concentration. This is difficult in the church setting since everyone knows one another and desires to fellowship and chat in between their turns to be on stage. However, all players can easily be reminded that to watch their fellow actors is a courtesy, and to pray for them is a privilege.

2. Feel your part. Stanislavski wrote in *An Actor Prepares,* "Feel your part and instantly all your inner chords will harmonize, your whole bodily apparatus of expression will begin to function. Therefore, we have found the first and most important master—FEELING. Unfortunately, it is not tractable nor willing to take orders. Since you cannot begin your work unless your feelings happen to function of their own accord, it is necessary for you to have recourse to some other master. Who is it? IMAGINATION!" This quote captures the essence of acting from inner motivation. Have your cast remember this rule: An external production is formal, cold, and pointless if it is not motivated from within. *Do more than just recite lines!*

3. Recall your emotions. After establishing the significance of performing with feeling and reminding the cast that feelings cannot be ordered to appear magically, help them by suggesting that they start to use their imaginations to recall certain emotions that will arouse desired feelings. Remind them:

A. THE ABILITY TO BE AN ACTOR IS BASED ON THE CAPACITY TO FEEL.

B. ACTORS ARE NOT DIVIDED BY TYPES—THEIR DIFFERENCES ARE MADE BY THEIR INNER QUALITIES.

C. EVERY PERSON HAS WITHIN THEM GOOD AND BAD. THEREFORE, ANY OF US COULD PLAY A VICTIM AS WELL AS A VILLAIN.

D. AS HUMANS OUR FEELINGS ARE AFFECTED BY OUR SURROUNDINGS. LIKEWISE THE SET, COSTUMES, AND LIGHTS WILL GREATLY AFFECT THE ACTOR'S ABILITY TO FEEL.

4. Raise your feelings. Stress to the cast that understanding they must act with feeling is not enough. If they do not learn how to summon their feelings, they'll wind up going at them directly, which is disastrous. That can be compared to a woman who tries to give birth to a full-grown man instead of a precious little boy. Imagine the missed joy and the added stress! Also, envision harvesting a garden of vegetables or flowers without ever having planted seeds (or without the process of water and sun). Impossible! Just the same, we musn't have contrived feelings on stage, or the audience will know. Therefore, acting is just like birthing or planting. "How do I plant these feelings?" You don't! They're already there if you're alive. On stage we merely arrive at certain feelings by drawing from personal experiences.

(As an exercise, ask for all cast members to name an emotional experience they have had, but to first identify the emotion felt. Whether they tell of the love they felt at the birth of a child or the pain they experience at the loss of one, search for that "look" in their eyes as they share their story. Afterwards, review certain stories that were shared and the effect they had on those who listened or witnessed the memory. The witnesses too may have had similar memories stirred up in them as they listened, which is exactly the effect a cast should have on their audience. But in addition, this ability to bear witness to another's emotion is also what enables the actor to portray a character and travel his emotional journey very realistically. In essence, the actor is sympathizing with his character.

5. Hunt for your emotions. If raising feelings is still a foreign concept to your cast, or if a few of them truly appear to have only one level of responsiveness, then encourage them to "hunt" for their feelings. This concept will especially help the male cast members as they compare the sport of hunting wild game to the idea of hunting for their emotions!

6. Don't stop! An actor who "puts the brakes" on his feelings once they begin to flow to an audience, is like a singer who misses her high note! (Have the cast imagine that they are spectators at the crucifixion of Jesus of Nazareth—one Man, divinely human, taking on the entire weight of all the world's sins, past and future; dying the most painfully slow death possible. Would watching this have been an emotional experience? Did Jesus stoicly brave His way through that dark day because He knew He would soon rest again by the right hand of God? Or did His humanity prevail and cause Him to question God's purposes for the unbearable pain and shame? Whether or not He was able to keep sight of His holy objectives, His humanity was with him to the end as he shouted such pleas as, "My, God, why hast thou forsaken me?" Surely watching this would have been emotional for the spectator, but never more emotional and dramatic than Jesus' own personal turmoil—emotional, human turmoil that could not be altered even by His holiness. If it had been altered, would His great act of love mean as much to us today?)

7. Communicate on stage. After finding your feeling, communicate onstage with the others who have found theirs. This is when your play will be complete. If every actor successfully finds his or her own feelings, but fails to communicate with the other actors who have also located theirs, then the process again is incomplete and defeated. Should an actor concentrate wholly on his own performance and then take a break while the next actor who speaks convincingly recites his lines? No! Acting is not a series of repeating one's lines, despite their believability. "If actors really mean to help the attention of a large audience they must make every effort to maintain an uninterrupted exchange of feelings, thoughts, and actions among themselves . . . May we see disappear forever the actor's blank eye, his immobile face and brow, his dull voice, speech without inflection, his contorted body with its stiff backbone and neck, his wooden arms, hands, finger, legs in which there is no motion, his slouching gait and painful mannerisms!"—Stanislavski.

8. Avoid tension. The actor who has perfected his craft and discovered his feelings will still miss the mark if he is physically tense. Muscular tension interferes greatly with emotional experience. As an exercise, choose one cast member, preferably a man, to lift a large, heavy object within the room. The larger the better, even if he can only bend to budge one side of the object. As he lifts, test the quickness of his five senses by asking him to respond to the following as fast as he can:

1. Quickly divide 112 by 4. (If he seems baffled then ask him to recall the exact number of buttons on his shirt.)
2. Describe the taste of a Thanksgiving turkey.
3. Describe the feel of a football.
4. Sing your favorite hymn.
5. Describe the smell of burnt toast.

As the actor collapses from exhaustion or retreats with embarrassment at his inability to think while holding the object, remind your cast that this response was expected. The actor should respond by being too consumed with the physical tension of holding the object to be able to use his memory recall. Therefore, failure to be relaxed on stage will also be the direct cause of an actor's inability to find his true inner feelings and objectives.

9. Relax and Warm up before each rehearsal and performance. Urge actors always to warm up each part of their physical bodies before taking the stage. Also exercising facial and vocal muscles is necessary to loosen the actor's muscles. (See Chapter 12, Opening Night, for more extensive warm up ideas.)

10. Character quiet times are a must. This is the culmination of all the acting techniques and preparations suggested thus far. Coaching the cast to learn their lines, find their feelings, and relax their bodies is all anticlimactic unless the process is ended with prayer and a true search for character purpose. Having actors review the questions at the bottom of their Discovering Your Character's Objectives worksheet will be most helpful in determining their spiritual influence on their audience. This character quiet time is the perfect mental preparation for the deeper task that awaits them as they take the stage, and praying for God's leadership will also allow the Holy Spirit to gain full creative control of their performance.

In conclusion, if these creative disciplines to Stanislavski are called "Method Acting," then to the Christian performer who adds the elements of prayer and spiritual reflection, they can be referred to as "Christian Method Acting" or "Creative Christian Character Development." A performance that is motivated from within may be needful, but one that is also motivated by the Holy Spirit indwelling our Christian souls delivers the essence of the human spirit which so desperately needs edification, as well as creative expression.

11

Publicity and Budgeting

Imagine a dinner theatre production that has been designed and rehearsed for months. The actors have successfully given life to what was once just numerous pages of written words. Technical crews have painstakingly matched each moment of the play with the proper visual and material effects. The meal, once merely a menu, is now hot and waiting to be dished onto the plates, and the director's job is done. But was it done well? What if after all that preparation only ten people come to see the play? Can you imagine the disappointment the cast and crew would experience? It could be compared to a child who sits alone at his extravagant birthday party, all because his mother forgot to mail the invitations. Or what about the groom who waits at the church for his bride, and then realizes he forgot to ask for her hand in marriage?

Publicity should never be viewed as less important than the other dinner theatre committees, or skimped on simply because its crew will not begin its work until late in the production process. Likewise, proper budgeting cannot be forsaken before a production is underway, or the entire dinner theatre will be built on a shaky foundation that inevitably will crumble, all as a result of poor planning. Budgeting and publicity can be thought of as first the cornerstone, and then the rooftop of your production. Therefore, this chapter will assist your group by offering specific successful ways to fully discharge the advantages of each.

Budgeting For Your Production

CATERER	COSTUMES	NURSERY
PLATES/CUPS/ETC.	LIGHT RENTALS	SOUND RENTALS
FILM DEVELOPMENT	CENTERPIECES	SCAFFOLD RENTAL
STAGE FLOWERS	STAGE CONSTR.	PRINTING PAPER
PRINTING COSTS	VIDEO TAPES	STAGE PROPS
MAKEUP	PUBLICITY COST	(MISC. ITEMS)

The above categories, and any others your play requires, should be budgeted for before your rehearsals begin. Whatever your budget or church budget allows for dramatic productions, begin by projecting expected costs in each of the mentioned categories. There is no reason why ticket sales cannot completely cover every one of these expenses. However, you may need to be fronted some money since your play's expenses naturally will come before its ticket income or profit. If your dinner theatre is church funded, the major expenses such as costumes, caterer, serviceware, etc., can all be purchased on an account and paid for at a later date by your church financial secretary. Also remember that every church has a tax I.D. # that makes their purchases tax exempt. This will save your church production lots of unnecessary costs.

Your budgeting needs will change with each play you produce. For instance, *The Incentive* and *The Healing* are both present-day plays, so costumes can be collected from each actor's personal wardrobe, thus eliminating the need for a costume allowance. But, supplying adequate stage lighting for *The Healing* will be a financial challenge if you do not have free access for borrowing lighting equipment. In this case, lighting would be a larger cost to accommodate than say, costumes, which again are not a necessity for this play.

Depending on how much money you need to recoup on the above categories of your dinner theatre production, plan for at least two perform-ances: a Saturday-night and a Sunday-matinee performance. If your ticket price is $5 and your caterer charges you $3.50 per plate, then you'll profit $1.50 for each person who attends. If you need to recoup $500 in play expenses, then you'll need to sell 333 tickets to break even (remember that after the caterer is paid you'll only profit $1.50 per head). If your auditorium has a seating capacity of just over 100 people, then you'll need to plan for three performances in order to sell these 333 tickets and break even. More performances will need to be scheduled to make a profit. If your auditorium seats less than this, then either plan for more perform-ances or spend less money on your play's production.

As a good rule, only spend money for your play that you can recoup directly through ticket sales. Use this guide to calculate how much money you'll have to spend on your production:

1. **TICKET PRICE MINUS CATERER PER PLATE PRICE = PROFIT PER PERSON**
2. **PROFIT PRICE X AUDITORIUM CAPACITY X NUMBER OF PER-FORMANCES = TOTAL DINNER THEATRE PROFIT (ALLOWANCE).**

If your ticket price is $5 and your caterer's per plate price is $4, then you'll make only $1.00 profit per seat. If your building can seat and feed 300 people and you are planning on three performances, then you'll have $900 to bank or spend on your play's expenses. This all is contingent, of course, on if you sell out all three performances. Alternatives for making more money include (a) raising your ticket price, (b) holding more performances, or (c) finding a cheaper caterer.

Publicity

Approximately four weeks before the play's first performance, the director should hold a special meeting with the publicity coordinator (and the publicity crew if one has been appointed). Items discussed should be:

1. What specific date tickets go on sale
a. Tickets should be sold for three weeks prior to the performance. The date by which your caterer needs a head count to begin preparing his food is the date that tickets should go off sale.
2. Preparing advertising/flyers before tickets go on sale
a. These are the 8½ x 11 flyers that will be distributed to advertise your play.
3. Discussing what information should go on the flyers
a. See sample flyer to follow from *The Healing*.
4. Find a graphic artist to design flyers / tickets / programs.
a. A friend with a computer can handle this, if you cannot.
5. Choosing a theme color for printing of flyers/tickets/program
a. A color that ties in with the theme or title of your play
6. Which local areas of interest should display the flyers
a. Check in your area Yellow Pages for local churches, schools, stores, merchants, etc.
7. Who will distribute ads to these locations?
a. The Publicity coordinator should have responsibility for this area.
8. Contacting media with publicity pictures: radio/TV/newspaper
a. Free ads from local TV talk shows, TV community calendars, radio stations offering free ads for community or church, newspaper ads and free newspaper editorial write-ups
9. General mailouts to community or church visitors.
a. Previous church visitors, community civic organizations, and social clubs that may wish to purchase multiple tickets or sponsor an entire table
10. Ads in your church's organization's bulletins
a. Weekly newsletter, weekly bulletins, hallway bulletin boards displaying your publicity shots/photos.

FIRST BAPTIST CHURCH OF DONELSON'S DINNER THEATRE PRESENTS

THE HEALING
THE HEALING

BY LAURA HARRIS SMITH

heal (hēl) v. 1. to restore or return. 2. to mend or set right.

SATURDAY, SEPTEMBER 22, 1990 - 7:00 PM
SUNDAY, SEPTEMBER 23, 1990 - 12:30 PM

$5.00 TICKET PRICE INCLUDES A CATERED DINNER AND PLAY

TICKETS MUST BE PURCHASED BY SEPTEMBER 19TH

nursery available for children - birth thru 3 years at a cost of
$3.00/1 child, $5.00/2 children, $7.50/3 children
nursery reservation must be made and paid for by september 19th .
parents are responsible for feeding nursery age children prior to arrival.

CONTACT DREW ANN BORSOS OR STEPHANIE HARMON

883-2339

FIRST BAPTIST CHURCH DONELSON
2526 LEBANON ROAD

THE HEALING
THE HEALING

"Confess your trespasses to one another, and pray for one another, that you
may be healed." James 5:16

The previous flyer can serve as a helpful aid in creating your own press release. Instead of using the definition of "Heal" for the teaser, you may wish to give a brief description of the play's content. If you can arrange volunteers to provide childcare for your event, then note on your flyer that childcare will be free. This is sure to increase ticket sales from parents with small children. Creating these flyers with all the necessary information on your play will greatly reduce the many calls and questions you'll receive and will provide an inexpensive boost in generating the excitement you need to increase ticket sales.

Since the director will be overloaded with last-minute preparations for the play, the publicity coordinator will have a fresh outlook on handling these responsibilities. The director will be involved, especially in the creative aspects, but allowing the publicity coordinator to assume these tasks will insure that the play is advertised to its fullest potential.

What would happen if your dinner theatre was not well-publicized? All your hard work would have been in vain. And what if you had never budgeted well to begin with? Your production would either be bankrupt a month into rehearsals, or at the play's end you would discover a huge debt hanging over your head. Publicity is sure to bring in money, and budgeting assures the equal distribution of it. So give adequate and equal focus to both, for to abandon either will greatly debilitate your entire dinner-theatre production.

12

Opening Night!

Opening Night. Those two words can send a rush of adrenaline through any performer's body, leaving him ecstatic and paralyzed all at once. Opening night signifies that the time and talents of many have been offered, accepted, and employed. It indicates the end of one chapter and the long-awaited beginning of another. "To everything there is a season, a time to every purpose under Heaven: A time to be born, and a time to die; a time to plant and a time to pluck up that which is planted . . ." On and on the verses read in Ecclesiastes 3, each teaching the significance of life's various seasons. Of course, the Bible need not ever be amended, but perhaps the performers' translation of this passage would be: "There is a time to rehearse and a time to enact." In short, Opening Night announces the end of practice, and the beginning of performance.

In spite of this completion, all endings mark the beginning of another starting point. And every starting point initiates a new labor; some new activity that must be embraced and maintained. Regardless of who you are, or for what purpose you have started your dinner theatre, Opening Night creates a universal surge of nervous tension and excitement. Many believe that a good case of stage fright provides the actor with two assurances. One: he is alive. And two, his performance may actually be enhanced by the extra flow of adrenaline his mind and body are receiving. Still, this is little consolation to the inexperienced actor. All he knows is that his heartbeat and visits to the restroom have increased dramatically while his confidence level simultaneously wanes.

If left unassisted, this actor's performance may certainly be affected, and not for the better. Nervous energy is normal, but there is no reason why it cannot be fastened down and taught to converge with peace and direction. This is the director's responsibility, although the temptation may be to consider his or her job done, and to sit down and eat a well-deserved dinner. Directors can certainly stop to enjoy the fruits of their laboring on

Opening Night, as long as they realize that their "laboring" is not complete until the cast is emotionally, physically, and spiritually primed to perform.

Emotional Preparation

First, your dinner theatre's actors and actresses will arrive early for their makeup calls and spend an hour or so in their dressing rooms getting into costume and makeup. These tedious activities will keep them mentally occupied until they are dressed and waiting for the show to begin. This sudden idle time is usually when nerves have an opportunity to flare, but if the cast is refocused into other activities, their tension will taper, or may even be eliminated.

To begin with, reward your cast by providing for them a peaceful atmosphere in which to dress. Often, some cast members will want to bring music or even small televisions into the dressing rooms, but this should not be allowed. Distractions may greatly disturb the other cast members, and it would be unfair to those who thrive on peace and quiet. Also, if your dinner theatre is located in a church or some alternate facility, you may find yourself having to dress in preschool/nursery rooms or classrooms. Make every effort to transform the rooms (only one for men and only one for women) with quick access to the stage with assisted entrances from the stage manager, and to supply them with mirrors and easy accesses to restrooms. On hand for free use by the actors should be stage makeup, but also other unpredictable necessities such as aspirin, tissues, combs, deodorant, and hair spray. This way, should they discover they have forgotten something, they are less likely to become frantic and want to return home to get it. Keep ice water on hand throughout the performances, too, since the cast will always be ready for a quick refreshment.

In addition to supplying the cast with pleasant, well-stocked dressing areas, the director should check in on them as they are dressing to assist them in any way. As they appear to be finishing their dressing routines, the time is appropriate to distribute his or her notes of thanks to the cast and crew. Since they'll be waiting for the play to begin and trying to battle their nerves, notes of praise will ease their minds and give them a sense of accomplishment, despite the results of their performances. Even though they will receive applause from their audience, a note of appreciation from the director should not be neglected, regardless of when they're distributed.

As the cast is waiting backstage, the house will be opened and guests will begin to be ushered in and seated. Every dinner theatre committee is now functioning at its fullest capacity, preparing for the meal and show to begin. Friendly house managers are greeting guests and checking guest lists while the guests they've seated are reading over their informative programs. The technical crews are running lighting and sound checks. The stage manager is going over his or her cue book to double check each entrance and exit. Prop managers are busy, counting props and placing them within easy reach of all the cast members. The kitchen managers are scurrying about in the kitchen, piloting cups and plates like they are directing traffic. Slowly, the caterer lifts the lid off of a steaming container of his delicious food, and as the very first plate is dipped, the dinner theatre has officially commenced.

The cast, with trays in hand, now flows through the audience in full character, serving the food and greeting the guests. If anyone in the cast was not emotionally prepared before this, the audience interaction will certainly complete the process for that actor or actress. Serving the meal and filling drinks should take about fifteen minutes total. Then, with the guests left to enjoy their meals, the cast can return backstage and continue preparing themselves to perform.

Physical Preparation

The physical exercise provided by serving so many guests will no doubt get the cast's blood flowing, but it may actually leave them quite hyper. Again, adrenaline rushes are beneficial in adding that "edge" to your actors' performances, but the effects are unpredictable on the body. Remember in Chapter 10 how the effects of a tense body on emotional recall were examined? Actors could not lift heavy objects and use their five senses simultaneously. Likewise, since your cast members may have overexerted themselves physically by serving, they need to regroup before performing.

Assemble the cast members and have them each find a space they can relax in within the sound of your voice. Begin with floor exercises. Any floor exercises are fine, as long as they involve stretching, which of course is effective in soothing and loosening the actors' tense muscles. After stretching, next have the actor curl into a ball with his face to the floor. Releasing one vertebra at a time, the actor can then rise slowly, building his way to a standing position with arms, hands, and head still hanging. Once vertical, the head can be raised and then rolled from side to side, rotating the neck. With eyes closed, facial exercises that stretch the jaw and mouth are vital to relaxing the actor's face. End the exercises by accompanying these movements with sound. This is recommended since the actor's voice will also need preparation. Suggest that the actors stretch their facial muscles while releasing long vowel sounds, exaggerating the muscle movements needed to produce the following sounds:

continuous: A-A-E-E-I-I-O-O-U-U-("Ay-eee-i-oh-ooo")

Spiritual Preparation

With the cast still assembled, direct their attention to discussing the importance of the task that lies ahead of them. Regardless of your play's message and theme, many lessons and morals will be discovered by the audience since, as a rule, audiences always share the emotional journeys of the characters they watch. Because the theatre can provide a format in which the viewers' lives are acted out, teaching is always in progress, whether the audience learns from the characters' victories or from their mistakes. Therefore, any play, secular or religious, contains teachable moments, and the cast performing that play has the spiritual responsibility to seize every teachable moment possible.

As suggested in Chapter 10 on the Discovering Your Character's Objectives worksheet, reviewing the spiritual questions before each performance helps each character maintain his or her clear objective throughout the play. In addition to this character quiet time, leading the cast through a related devotional can be the perfect ending to the long road on which you've all just traveled. Ecclesiastes 7:8 reads, "The end of a thing is better than its beginning, and the patient in spirit is better than the proud in spirit." Reflect with the cast on the very first rehearsal you had. Recall each and every difficulty you faced and every hurdle you successfully vaulted. Remind them that their patience and diligence will soon be rewarded and that they've put together a wonderful production.

Finally, lead your cast in prayer. They deserve it. Spiritual preparation is no less important than emotional and physical preparation because all actors are merely human, spiritual beings. Pray for each actor's performance and for any special needs within the cast. Close by asking that God prepare the hearts and minds of the waiting audience, for they will be the recipients of your labor of love.

Opening Night. You will be excited for its coming and yet comforted by its passing. After Opening Night, your production will seem to coast on auto-pilot, as you all reap the rewards of your months of hard work. Regardless of the size of your cast, your play, or your crowd, it will be a significant evening for all to remember for a long while. In fact, no other show can match its level of intensity, except maybe the Opening Night of your next production!

At long last, good luck and congratulations on your worthy decision to establish your dinner theatre. Your attempts and efforts already equal instant accomplishment, and God is pleased. So relish the emotions and savor the sentiments that will linger long after your first curtain call is over. Your dinner theatre may be planning several performances, but never forget there is only one *OPENING NIGHT!*

THE INCENTIVE

by
Laura Harris Smith

SYNOPSIS

The Acklen family has a serious problem—themselves! Spoiled rotten daughters *Kathleen, Cassandra,* and *Kelly Ann* are all grown and yet still living at home with their husbands and families (Kelly Ann is not married, of course, because no man will have her). Kathleen, the eldest and loudest, is the widowed mother of three teenage, boy-crazy girls. Elegant Cassandra, the middle and most immodest daughter, is married to *Owen Beacham* and with the exception of their adopted teenage son, Ben, they are childless (which, of course, is *not* her fault). Kelly Ann, the baby, has yet to find a man who is "good enough" for her, so she remains at home, without a job, in search of a lavender piano to match her bedroom. The entire family is greedy, selfish, unhappy, and extremely money-hungry. Quite content to carry on this way, they do so until their widowed mother, *Gwendolyn Acklen* (a godly woman whose character was not changed by the fortune left to her by her late husband) decides to force them to change. Of course, they don't make a habit of listening to her, but since she controls the family assets, they decide to take heed.

Set in the small Georgia city of Gibsonville, Gwen secretly calls upon the services of *Lillian Laraby,* attorney at law, a friend whom she knows has her family's best interests at heart. That Thanksgiving night, together, they plan a "departure" for Gwen (which the family comically mistakes for her death), after which a fictitious last will and testament is heard by the family. The hilarious "video will," that is actually viewed on stage, allows the audience to experience the family's surprise as Gwen notifies them that she is leaving $1 to be divided among the three girls (and, of course, they fight over the extra penny!). Lillian has been employed to monitor them for one year and if they alter their behavior, Gwen promises they will receive their full inheritances.

The plot springs forward as the months pass by, and we eavesdrop on the family's sluggish progress. Although the will provides the original incentive for the family to learn to love one another as they should, they gradually change by their own free "will." By the time Gwen re-enters on the next Thanksgiving Day, Kathleen has become the image of her mother, a loving single parent of three daughters. Cassandra and Owen's marriage has been mended and enhanced by the birth of a baby boy—and Kelly Ann is engaged to be married to a local piano salesman, who, although he is poor, loves her and provides her with a lavender piano.

The Incentive, a heartwarming comedy, devotes unique attention to the sensitive issues of adoption, infertility, marital disharmony, teenage dating, the love of money, and the backslidden Christian, proving how one woman's faith can change an entire family for the better—all with a good dose of laughter.

SETTING

The entire play takes place in the home of Gwendolyn Acklen, otherwise known as Acklen Manor. The play spans one year of time, and is set in the town of Gibsonville, a small town in Southern Georgia. The play begins on Thanksgiving Day, 1988, on a Thursday. It ends on Thanksgiving Day, 1989.

CHARACTERS

Gwendolyn Ann Acklen—58, from Gibsonville, Georgia. She is small, stout, and always pleasant. The mother of three girls, she has been a widow since she was 38 years old. She is patient, wise, and a woman of strong Christian faith. She has been left with a large fortune.

Kathleen Acklen Howard—35, also from Gibsonville. She is tall, slender, and very authoritative. The oldest of the Acklen daughters, she has three daughters herself. She was left a widow at age 28, when her husband, Murray, died. She and her daughters live with her mother.

Cassandra Acklen Beacham—32, from Gibsonville. She is beautiful and graceful and she knows it. Known to be snobbish, she is the middle Acklen daughter. She has been married for seven years to Owen Beacham, and after two unsuccessful years of trying to have a child, they adopted an eight-year-old boy. They reside at Acklen Manor.

Kelly Ann Acklen—27, from Gibsonville. She is petite and the last of the Acklen daughters. The "baby" in all ways, she is spoiled, arrogant, yet very cute. She is still single and still lives at Acklen Manor.

Marilyn Howard—16, is Kathleen's eldest daughter. She is energetic, youthful, and completely preoccupied with the subject of driving.

Rebecca Howard—14, is Kathleen's second daughter. She is shy and quiet, yet boy crazy nonetheless. On occasion, she is whiny.

Gracie Howard—13, is Kathleen's youngest daughter. She also is a typical "baby" and is absolutely adorable. Gracie is already a compulsive shopper.

Owen Beacham—34, also from Gibsonville. Owen is handsome enough, yet unsure of himself. Being married to Cassandra has not helped his insecurity; in fact, he rarely stands up to her bossiness. Instead, he tries to make peace and do what she says. Owen is a hard worker and a loving husband and father.

Benjamin Beacham—13, from Nashville, Tennessee. Adopted at age eight by Owen and Cassandra, he is a mild-mannered young man. Having lived in a children's home, Ben is most appreciative of his family, yet is not concerned with acting rich as they do.

Lesley Kelly—30, from Gibsonville. He is honest and mild-tempered, yet a bit awkward. He is in love with Kelly Ann Acklen and wishes to marry her. The owner of a piano store, he does not make much money, but is very happy.

Lillian Laraby—32, from Gibsonville. Lillian is an ambitious young attorney who is already a partner in a local law firm. She is a long-time friend of the Acklen family and attended school and college with Cassandra Acklen.

Wilson Foster—41, from Northern Georgia. He is loud, boisterous, and often deafening. He is pastor at Gwendolyn Acklen's church.

Miriam Foster—35. The wife of Rev. Foster, she is a typical pastor's wife. Hospitable and sweet, she smiles constantly. She is the mother of three children.

Cory Foster—16, Rev. Foster's son. Cory is tall, handsome, and timid. He likes Rebecca Howard.

(non-speaking roles: Two Foster daughters, ages four and infant. Also needed: Cassandra's newborn child.)

ACT ONE

The entire family is gathered in the living room/dining room of Acklen Manor. It is Thanksgiving Day, 1988. The Acklen family is slow to be seated, since they are all busy with other activities. At first, the family appears to be happy, but soon they reveal their typical argumentative behavior. As Gwendolyn persuades each of them to come to dinner, they reluctantly do so, treating this Thanksgiving meal is if it were any other.

Scene One

Gwen: (enters carrying a tray of sliced turkey) Why, Owen, you have carved a beautiful Thanksgiving turkey! Come see everyone. Come see this beautiful plate of turkey that Owen has carved!

Kathleen: (moving toward table) Oh, Mother, don't fuss over Owen like that. He may have spent ten minutes carving that turkey, but I spent all day yesterday thawing it, thirty minutes stuffing it, and five hours basting it.

Kelly Ann: (moving toward table) That's right, Mother. Besides, that new electric carver could cut the turkey all by itself.

Cassandra: (at table from beginning) Would you just listen to yourselves? It's obvious that both of *you* are jealous of *me* because I'm the only Acklen daughter with a husband present at the Thanksgiving table for seven years in a row.

(All three girls begin to argue loudly)

Gwen: Girls! Girls!!! (They are finally quiet) Thank you. I will remind you that today is Thanksgiving and that this is Thanksgiving dinner. If the three of you cannot find anything to be thankful for, then at least be grateful that you have a tolerant mother. Now, call your children and let's all be seated.

Kathleen: (screaming) Marilyn, Rebecca, Gracie . . . D-I-N-N-E-R!!!

Cassandra: Benjamin dear, have you washed your hands?

Ben: Yes, Mother.

Cassandra: Yes, but, did you scrub under your nails? Let me see those hands. I do believe it's time for another manicure, Benjamin.

Owen: Cassandra, please! Don't treat Ben that way. He's a boy, not a girl.

Kathleen: That's right, Cassandra. Remember, Sister dear, *I* got the girls. (yells loudly to them) Speed it up, will you?

Cassandra: I know he's a boy, Owen. But he still has hands, and all hands need to be manicured appropriately.

Owen: Cassandra, (stands) this boy will not have another manicure. You know we have already discussed this.

Kelly Ann: We *all* know. We couldn't help but overhear your *discussion* night before last. It kept us all awake!

Cassandra: Oh, Kelly Ann, what could you possibly understand about the responsibilities of children. You're not even married!

Kelly Ann: Well, watching the two of you it's no wonder!

Gracie: Grandmother, may we please eat? I'm famished.

All children: Yeah! Let's eat.

Gwen: Of course, my dears, we will eat now. But first, we must all think of one thing for which we are thankful. Then, after we have thanked God for those blessings, we will eat. Gracie, you and your sisters go first, followed by your mother. Kelly Ann, you'll then tell us something you are thankful for. Owen, Ben and Cassandra, you'll be next and then, I'll go last. (she sits).

Gracie: Well, I'm thankful that I turned thirteen this year, because for a while I was the only one around here who wasn't a teenager. I'm also pleased that I was accepted into the Teen Social League because that will grant me my very own, personal shopping account at Bloomingdale's!

Rebecca: Well, I'm still a year older than you and for that, I am thankful. I am also thankful that mother has agreed to let me start car-dating this year!

Marilyn: Mom! You didn't let me car-date until I was fifteen!

Kathleen: Becca, I did not say you could car-date with just anyone. I said I would consider it only if it was with that nice young boy at your grandmother's church. What is his name?

Rebecca: (sighs) His name is Cory.

Gwen: Oh, Becca! Do you mean Rev. Foster's son?

Rebecca: Yes, Grandmother.

Gwen: Oh, I'm so pleased. He certainly is handsome—and tall!

Rebecca: Well, he hasn't even asked me out yet, so don't say anything, please.

Gwen: All right. Marilyn, do you have something you're thankful for?

Marilyn: Yes, of course. I'm thankful for many things including my sisters and my mother, my aunts and my grandmother. But most of all, I am so glad that I passed my driver's test. Now, mother can buy me that new Jag!

Ben: Hey, Marilyn, that's great! Now you can chauffeur all of us around!

Kelly Ann: Congratulations, Marilyn! I just can't believe you're old enough to drive already! Well, I, like Marilyn, am thankful for my sisters, Cassandra and Kathleen, and their families. I am also thankful for my mother, whose fortune allows all of us to live in the same house without a care in the world!

Kathleen: If you don't have a care it's because you don't have a job. You skipped over me; it's my turn. Let's see, I am thankful for my daughters, despite the stress they cause me. I suppose I am thankful for my two younger sisters. And Mother, I know I say this every Thanksgiving, but I am most thankful to you for your help with the girls, even all these years after Murray's death.

Gwen: It's true what they say, you know.

All: What's that?

Gwen: A mother's work is never done!

Cassandra: Well, I'll second that. Owen, it's your turn.

Owen: Oh, I'm thankful for a beautiful wife. I have to be honest and say that I do wish we didn't argue as much as we do . . .

Cassandra: Owen!

Owen: Oh yes, Dear, well, let's see, I am thankful for all of you, and for a good job, and for a fine son like Ben. Go ahead, Son.

Ben: OK. I am grateful for Mom and Dad and Grandmother Gwen. I am glad that I have a warm bed, and so much food to eat. I am glad that I live with people who love me, and for a grandmother who takes me to church. I guess I am most thankful for my cousins, Marilyn, Rebecca, and Gracie. I guess you're the only sisters I will ever have!

Cassandra: Oh, Ben, I'm sorry that we haven't been able to give you a little brother or sister of your own. Of course (to Owen), *that isn't my fault.*

Owen: Now, Cassandra, don't start, please. We don't know whose fault it is that we can't have a child. Anyway, neither of us should blame each other. We should be thankful we're a family.

Cassandra: Thankful?! Thankful?!!?!! You want me to be thankful for this self-centered, egotistical, pathetic excuse of a family?

Owen: Well, (laughs a short, nervous laugh), yes.

Cassandra: You listen to me, Owen Beacham, it's turning my hair gray living in the same house with all of them, and you have the audacity to ask me to be thankful?!? I'll tell you what would make me thankful. (grabs large basket of rolls, dumps them onto table and begins filling the basket with spoonfuls from each platter). Dinner for one and an Excedrin would make me thankful! (As she exits, Owen and Ben follow to comfort her.)

Kelly Ann: Boy, she sure is sensitive lately.

Kathleen: Kelly Ann, pipe up until you get a husband. (leaves to find Cassandra)

Kelly Ann: (stands) I have been reminded one too many times today that I'm husbandless. You all seem to think that I don't want to be married, when the truth is I just can't find anyone who is good enough for me. Oh! This has turned out to be the worst Thanksgiving ever! (Leaves)

Marilyn: I do believe that Aunt Kelly Ann is right, Grandmother. Why don't we clear the table and try again later?

Gwen: Oh, Marilyn, I'm afraid you are right. Yes, honey that's fine. You girls gather the food and I'll clear the rest later.

(The girls do so and exit with the dishes.)

Scene Two

Gwen: (still at table) Well, I never got my turn. And I think I have got a lot to be thankful for. I am thankful for three beautiful daughters who, among them, have enough self-esteem to supply all of the world's introverts. I am also thankful for my four lovely grandchildren. I am thankful for my church, my home, and oh yes, my health. Well, despite all the bickering, a lot of thankfulness was expressed today, so I suppose I will have to give thanks to God all by myself. (prays) Our Heavenly Father, forgive this family for its numerous shortcomings. On this special Thanksgiving Day, I thank You for the way You have blessed all of us. Thank You especially for your Son. Help me to be a peacemaker, Lord. In Jesus' name I pray, Amen. (opens eyes and stands)

So, this is Thanksgiving Day. Hmmm. I think I am most thankful that Wendall is no longer here to see how this family carries on. January will be twenty years since I've seen you. (views a portrait of her late husband, wipes her eyes, then says angrily:) You left me with quite a handful when you died! Of course, you left me with quite a fortune too. (moves to portrait of Kathleen) Poor Kathleen. I know just how she feels being a young widow with three girls to raise. I imagine it's harder nowadays. The year Murray died she really had it rough. And that being the year that Cassandra married Owen only made things rougher. Cassandra was as happy as Kathleen was sad. But, she finished college and started teaching middle school. I suppose she's a good teacher. I just hope she has more patience with those school children than she does with her own. If you ask me, she yells too much. (moves to portrait of Cassandra) Then there's my beautiful Cassandra. If only she didn't know it. She's always trying to do what is "appropriate." Only I keep trying to tell her there is more to life than propriety. (Ben enters the room, but she does not notice.) I wish she was as concerned with her interior as she is with her exterior. She should be happy with a husband like Owen and a son like Ben.

Ben: Why do you think that Mother isn't happy?

Gwen: (startled) How long have you been listening, Benjamin?

Ben: Just long enough to make me think that something is wrong with my mom. Is there, Grandmother Gwen? I don't want her to be unhappy.

Gwen: Oh, Ben, you are so compassionate. And wise too! Why, at dinner tonight you were the only person who was thankful for all the right things. You couldn't care less about the Acklen money, could you?

Ben: Well, I suppose it's nice to be rich, but I haven't been that way long enough to know how to act rich! I can remember when I didn't know when I'd ever get a family. The children's home had enough money to keep me, but they couldn't be what I wanted the most—a family. I have that now, and for that I am thankful.

Gwen: Oh, Ben, adopting you was the wisest way that the Acklen money was ever spent! (They hug.) With all our money, the children's home assumed we could offer you everything. I fear now that you have been pulled into the middle of a very messed-up family.

Ben: Is my mother the problem?

Gwen: Oh no, my dear. Your mother is merely a symptom. I fear that I am the problem.

Ben: What do you mean?

Gwen: What I mean is, I have spared the rods and spoiled the children.

Ben: You mean, you've spoiled my mother, Aunt Kathleen, and Aunt Kelly Ann?

Gwen: Yes, Ben. But with the best of intentions. Your grandfather was so good to me. In fact, he spoiled me. We didn't have much when we first married, so when the Acklen Lumber Yard he started began to prosper, he built this place for me and made me a queen. The more that business grew, the more he spoiled me. Neither one of us had ever had money, so we did the only thing we knew how to do with it—enjoy it!

Ben: How did Grandfather die?

Gwen: It's not as if he died, Ben. One morning, he just never woke up. Dr. Curtis said his weak heart just failed him. He was a young man too, only 41. I was left with three little girls, ages fifteen, twelve, and seven.

Ben: Who ran the lumber yard?

Gwen: I did! For thirteen years I ran it from right here. We never had a son, and none of the girls wanted to inherit a lumber yard. Then, when your mother married your father, he offered to take it over for me. Owen has been running things for seven years now.

Ben: I know. He works really long hours too. Maybe that's why Mother is unhappy.

Gwen: No, I just don't think your mother knows how to be happy. Nobody can make you happy except you . . . and the Lord. You remember that, Ben. You know, you make your mother happy, Ben. She and your father tried for two years to have a child, and when that specialist told them they'd never have a child, they adopted you. They wanted a boy because, you see, Kathleen had given us all girls, and your mother knew how much I wanted a grandson.

Ben: But I'm not really your grandson.

Gwen: Benjamin Beacham! That hurt!

Ben: I'm sorry. It's just that, it's true.

Gwen: Ben, I love you. I know you love me. Therefore, you are family. You make me so happy, Ben. I know your Grandfather Acklen would have loved you too. He never had a son, so his first grandson inherits all of Acklen Lumber Yard—that's you!

Ben: Yes, but there's still plenty of time for Aunt Kelly Ann to get married and have the first real grandson.

Gwen: (chuckles) Don't hold your breath, Ben. No man in Gibsonville would have her as she is. No, there's no chance of her giving me another grandson anytime in the next decade.

Ben: Don't be upset, Grandmother. It sounds to me as if you did the best you could raising three kids all alone.

Gwen: Thank you, Ben.

Ben: Some people just don't know what they've got until it's gone.

Gwen: (Slowly she turns to him as if she has been struck with an idea.) Ben, say that again.

Ben: Some people just don't know what they've got until it's gone.

Gwen: Benjamin, you've given me an idea!

Ben: I have? I didn't mean to.

Gwen: That's what I love about you. Happy Thanksgiving, Ben.

Ben: Happy Thanksgiving, Grandmother. Good night.

Gwen: Good night, Dear.

Scene Three

(Ben leaves and Gwen approaches a desk, looking through an address book for a phone number. As she searches, she speaks aloud.)

Gwen: Dear Lord, here I go. Now if You don't want me to do this, please slam all the doors. And whatever You do, don't open a window, or I'll dive right in. Oh, here's that number. (She dials.) I do believe that I have found a way to get my family's attention and teach them a lesson. Yes, hello! Is this Lillian Laraby, attorney at law? Hello, Lillian Dear, this is Gwendolyn Acklen. (pause) Yes, well, it has been a long time. Dear, I am sorry to bother you on the Thanksgiving holiday, but... (She is interrupted as Kelly Ann enters the room.)

Kelly Ann: Mother, how long will you be on the phone? I have an urgent call to place.

Gwen: (into phone) Just a moment please. Kelly Ann, I have just placed this call. What could possibly be so urgent on a holiday evening?

Kelly Ann: I have decided that I must have a new piano. My old one just does not look appropriate in my room.

Gwen: Well, why not? What's wrong with it?

Kelly Ann: It's the wrong shade.

Gwen: Well, what *shade* should it be?

Kelly Ann: It should be lavender. I cannot be creative on such a drab-colored piano. I must have a lavender piano!

Gwen: Kelly Ann, I have never heard of a purple piano.

Kelly Ann: Not purple, Mother. Lavender. If I should fail to find a lavender piano, and you should choose to surprise me with one for Christmas, do not buy a purple one. Purple will still be the wrong shade. My room is lavender, so my piano must match. *Lavender.*

Gwen: Well, whatever kind of piano you want, there is no piano store open in Gibsonville tonight, so go to bed.

Kelly Ann: Yes, there is mother. It's the piano store on Melvin Street. I must call them before they close.

Gwen: The sooner you leave, the sooner I can finish, and the sooner you can have your piano. Now, I'll call you when I'm through.

Kelly Ann: All right, Mother. Just H-U-R-R-Y.

Gwen: (Kelly Ann leaves, and Gwen speaks to Lillian again.) I am so sorry, Lillian. Listen, I need to free this line, Dear. Would it be possible for you to pay me a visit tonight? It's regarding a legal matter, and I'll pay you extra since it's a holiday. (pause) Do you remember where we live? Of course, you do. Can you come now? (pause) Oh thank you, Dear! Oh, and don't ring the bell. Just knock softly, and I'll be waiting. Good-bye now. (hangs up) Well, that's one door opened. I guess I'd better tell Liberace that the line is clear. Kelly Ann? Kelly Ann!

Kelly Ann: Yes, Mother?

Gwen: You may use the phone now. I'm going upstairs. (points upwards)

Kelly Ann: Well, thank you finally. (dials directory assistance) Yes, may I please have the number of that piano store on Melvin Street? (pause) I don't know the name of the store, or I'd look it up myself, wouldn't I? (pause) Well, you must have seen it. It has a huge sign with big red letters that blink. Yes, I'll hold. (Long pause) Kelly's? Kelly's Piano Parlour? Yes, that's it! Well, isn't that just grand? I'm going to order a piano for myself from myself! (giggles) 472-2384. (slams phone—then picks up and dials again) Hello, this is Kelly Ann Acklen, and I want to . . . yes, this is *the* Kelly Ann Acklen. Why? Do I know you? (pause) Oh, I see. Well, I have never talked to my secret admirer before. Although, I've had many I am sure. You want what? (pause) Well, I don't know. I have never been on a blind date. You're not blind, are you? (pause) Good. You're not color blind either, are you? Good. Because I need a lavender piano delivered tonight. (pause) Oh, I see. Well, how long will it take for you to search for one? (pause) Oh, I see. (pause) Yes, well, I suppose one little date couldn't do any harm. Are you short? You sound short. (pause) Good, because I am, and I don't like short men. All right then, you may call on me. Good-bye. (hangs up) Being beautiful is such a burden! (sighs and then exits)

Scene Four

(Gwen re-enters—as she does there is a knock at the door, and she scurries to answer it before anyone hears.)

Gwen: Oh, Lillian, do come in!

Lillian: Hello, Mrs. Acklen. It's been a while since I've been here.

Gwen: Yes (taking her coat), I was thinking. It has been at least ten years, because it was when you and Cassandra were planning your college-graduation parties. And please, don't call me Mrs. Acklen anymore. Call me Gwendolyn.

Lillian: All right. I haven't really talked with Cassandra since college. How is she, and the others?

Gwen: Well, you know she and Owen were married two years after college, and a couple of years later they adopted a young boy named Benjamin.

Lillian: Well, I'm happy for them. With my schedule the way it is, I might never have a family.

Gwen: Now, Lillian, I am very proud of you. Even ten years ago, I knew you'd make a fine attorney. And here you are sitting before me, all grown up and a partner in a big law firm. At your age you should feel that is quite an achievement! Goodness knows, if just one of my daughters expressed such enthusiasm about anything, I would be delighted.

Lillian: Now, Mrs. Acklen—I mean Gwendolyn—your daughters are the center of local conversation. Every little girl in Gibsonville would like to be an Acklen daughter for a day.

Gwen: You're joking.

Lillian: Well, no. I've even wished that I could be an Acklen girl. I used to love visiting here. Sometimes I even pretended that you were my mother!

Gwen: Now, Lillian, you ought to thank our all-knowin' Lord that I am not. I am afraid I have failed miserably with all three of my girls.

Lillian: What ever do you mean? Is there something wrong?

Gwen: Lillian, yes. Yes, there *is* something wrong. One by one I brought three little, pink bundles home from the hospital. They were so sweet and thoughtful, all three of them. Somehow, all of them have been secretly taken from my home and replaced with three stingy, loud-mouthed, money-hungry snobs!

Lillian: (surprised) Why, Mrs. Acklen, I had no idea that things were that way. I am sorry. I wish I could help.

Gwen: But you can!

Lillian: How?

Gwen: You can help me get rid of all this.

Lillian: Wait a minute. You want me to help you get rid of your fortune?

Gwen: In a way, yes. I have this plan, you see, but it cannot be carried out alone. If my plan succeeds, my girls and their families will no longer be motivated by material possessions.

Lillian: I don't think I understand.

Gwen: I know, Dear. I am getting ahead of myself. Let me start from the beginning and explain why I've called upon your services on this holiday. You see, Lillian, my girls never had to work for what they wanted. I understand now that having enough money to give your children everything they could *ever* want is a mixed blessing. After Wendell died, I smothered the girls with gifts, letting them indulge themselves whenever I felt they were missing their father or even when they were not. Today, they still depend on money to bring them happiness. Honestly, I feel like this is my fault, and finally, I am going to correct the problem.

Lillian: What are you going to do?

Gwen: I'm going to leave them. Some people just don't know what they've got until it's gone, you know.

Lillian: You're going to leave? Well, other than making them miss you, that really won't do much good, will it?

Gwen: Lillian, what happens when a person dies?

Lillian: Why, you know the answer to that. It depends on whether or not they are a Christian.

Gwen: Yes, I'm sorry. What I meant was, what legal procedures follow the death of an individual with an estate the size of mine?

Lillian: Well, as soon as that person's attorney is officially notified, the attorney contacts the family, and arrangements are made for an execution of the last will and testament.

Gwen: Well, then, consider yourself officially notified.

Lillian: (stands) Wait a minute, are you suggesting that I help you fake your death?

Gwen: (laughs) Oh no, dear, I'm not a good-enough actress to pull that off, and besides, I could never deceive my family like that.

Lillian: Well then, why would you want your family to hear your will? Providing you have left your possessions to them, wouldn't that just be giving them what they want? More money?

Gwen: Aha! Not if I made them work for it first!

Lillian: Oh, Mrs. Acklen—I mean Gwendolyn—I'm not sure I understand all of this. If you don't want to fake your death, then you won't be deceased. And if you aren't deceased, your family, by law, cannot have access to your will. If you don't want to play dead, than what do you want?

Gwen: I want to live to see my daughters happy—really happy. With or without money. Lillian, is it possible that I could go away somewhere, and have you contact my family as an attorney, and explain to them that I am safe and well? You could tell them that I chose this time to go away, and in my absence I am leaving them responsible for my estate, *if* they meet all the requirements I establish.

Lillian: Requirements? So what you are suggesting is, that your family will not be able to have their inheritances until their behaviors change.

Gwen: Precisely. Of course, this isn't my real will. I'll have you draw up a pretend one!

Lillian: But, when would you return, and how would you know if they've improved?

Gwen: I would stay away for one year, and you could monitor their progress. I'll pay you very well, my Dear.

Lillian: Well, I wouldn't be telling them that you were dead, so I wouldn't be lying, and the will would not be notarized so I wouldn't be doing anything illegal. But, Gwendolyn, where will you go for an entire year? How will I know where to locate you with the progress reports?

Gwen: I haven't figured that out yet. But I will! Let me think here.

Lillian: (pause) May I say something?

Gwen: Of course, Dear.

Lillian: Well, as an attorney, I cannot accept a fee for doing this or it might misrepresent my firm.

Gwen: But, Lillian, I insist on compensating you for this. It will be a full year of work.

Lillian: Then may I name my price?

Gwen: You may.

Lillian: For one year you will compensate me by fulfilling an old dream of mine.

Gwen: What's that, Dear?

Lillian: Allow me to be an Acklen daughter for one year and come stay with me.

Gwen: Why, Lillian Laraby! You *are* cleverly creative! I like it. Let's do it!

Lillian: You can come whenever you're ready and we'll draw up this will.

Gwen: Is tonight too soon?

Lillian: I suppose not. It looks to me like I won't spend Thanksgiving alone after all!

Gwen: Good-bye for now.

Lillian: Good-bye, *Mother Acklen.* (she exits)

Scene Five

(It is the next morning. Kathleen enters wearing a robe and drinking coffee.)

Kathleen: Oh, the rest of these dishes were never cleared. Oh well, I'll leave them, and maybe we can have a successful post-Thanksgiving breakfast.

Gracie: (enters dressed) May I have an advance on my allowance?

Kathleen: How about "good morning, Mother"?

Gracie: (exits briefly, then re-enters) Good morning, Mother. May I have an advance on my allowance?

Kathleen: That's a small improvement. Where are your sisters?

Gracie: Oh, they've gone driving.

Kathleen: How much do you need? (gets checkbook)

Gracie: I am not sure yet. I am going shopping with Mallory Jenkins, and I don't know how much she will buy yet!

Kathleen: What does that mean?

Gracie: It means that I can't let her outspend me!

Kathleen: All right, Dear, just record the amount in my checkbook later.

Gracie: Yes, Mother. Ta ta!

Kathleen: Ta ta. (sips coffee) Ta ta? Did I say Ta ta?

Cassandra: (enters carrying a large box of winter sweaters) Can't find anyone else to talk to but yourself, Kathleen?

Kathleen: Oh, good morning, Cassandra. I see you are back to your normal self again.

Cassandra: If you are referring to last night's dinner conversation, I hardly think that was my fault.

Kathleen: Whatever you say, Sassy Cassy.

(enter Kelly Ann dressed)

Kelly Ann: Are you arguing already this morning?

Cassandra: No. I refuse to let chatty Kathy insult me any further. (pause) Have either one of you seen Mother?

Kelly Ann: No, why?

Cassandra: When I passed by her room to get my winter sweaters, it appeared that she was gone already. In fact, her bed looked unslept in.

Kathleen: (has crossed to a desk to search for a note) I don't see a note saying when she will return. Hey, you don't suppose she got angry after dinner last night and decided to . . .

Kelly Ann: Decided to what?

Kathleen: To leave.

Owen: Good morning, Ladies.

Cassandra: Oh, Owen, have you heard? Mother's run away!

Owen: What?

Ben: Good morning, everyone.

Cassandra: Ben, when did you last see your grandmother?

Ben: Uh, I saw her last night. We had a talk.

Kathleen: Ben, did she say anything that would lead you to believe that she was upset?

Cassandra: Don't interrogate my Benjamin! (harshly to Ben) Ben, did she say anything that would lead you to believe she was upset?

Ben: Well . . .

All: Well, what?

Ben: Well, yes, she did. She's upset at all of us. And I don't blame her. But she does.

Kelly Ann: What?

Ben: She blames *herself* for the way this family behaves.

Cassandra: Oh dear. Oh dear! Oh dear!! You don't suppose Mother has decided to . . . punish herself?

Owen: Punish herself?

Kathleen: Cassandra, are you suggesting that our mother has . . . ?

Owen: Calm down everyone. Now, who saw her last?

Kelly Ann: I think I did.

Owen: Did she say anything unusual?

Kelly Ann: No. She just said, "I am going upstairs." (points upstairs)

(Suddenly everyone assumes that this meant Gwen was referring to going to heaven, and they become hysterical.)

Cassandra: Oh no, this is dreadful! (There is a knock at the door.)

Owen: Maybe that's her!

Cassandra: Oh, Owen, she lives here. She wouldn't knock! (Enter Lillian Laraby.)

Lillian: Hello, Cassandra.

Cassandra: (surprised) Oh, hello, Lillian. It's good to see you—only I'm afraid you have chosen a bad time for a visit. Our mother has run away from home, and we are afraid she is going to harm herself.

Lillian: I know, that's why I'm here.

Kelly Ann: Come in, Lillian. What do you know that we don't?

Lillian: Hello, everyone. Well, I know where your mother is, and she isn't going to harm herself.

All: (in mass confusion) Where? Is she all right? Where is she?

Lillian: Your mother has gone away. But she is all right. I am here as her attorney to allow you to hear her last will and testament.

Cassandra: But you said she was all right. Why do we need to hear her will?

Kelly Ann: (smiling) Did you say "will"?

Owen: Kelly Ann! Hello, I am Owen Beacham, Cassandra's husband. Would you please explain this to us? We are very much confused.

Lillian: I am sorry, everyone, but I have been hired by your mother to execute a will and nothing more.

Cassandra: I demand to know where my mother is!

Lillian: She is safe, and she's being cared for. Now if you'll let me play this, you will all understand things more clearly.

Kelly Ann: What's that?

Lillian: This is the last will and testament of Mrs. Gwendolyn Ann Acklen. If you don't have a video cassette recorder, we can move this meeting to my office.

Kathleen: Of course, we have one. It's over here.

(Everyone mumbles hysterically.)

Kathleen: All right, everybody, get a grip on it and sit down. You may begin, Miss Laraby.

Scene Six

(Everyone is seated around the television as Lillian begins the video tape.)

Gwen: (nervously into camera) Uh, hello. I-I, Gwendolyn Ann Acklen, being of sound mind, (aside) excuse me, is it sound mind or sound body? I'm sorry. I've never done this before. Could I have some iced tea? Whew! It's awfully hot in here. (takes a quick sip) I'm ready now. If you don't mind I'll just speak my mind and leave out the "thees" and "thous." (into camera again) Hello, family. This is your mother . . . and your grand-mother. Oh, I hope all of you are listening because I have something important to discuss with you. I have left you now, and you must all learn to live without me. (sips tea) Hey, this is good! (takes a long drink)

Cassandra: Oh, Owen! Look at her! She's gone senile! (hysterically) *Our mother has checked herself into a home for the senile!* (She collapses and Owen fans her.)

Kelly Ann: Is it hereditary?

Gwen: Now, where was I? Oh, I remember. You are all going to have to learn to live without me, and here is where you begin. This isn't going to be any ordinary will, so I suggest that you get comfortable and fasten your seat belts. Owen, you had better get Cassandra's fan. I'll begin with my daughters. Kathleen, Cassandra, and Kelly Ann. My years with you have been eventful and memorable, to say the least. Girls, I love you all dearly.

(Kathleen, Cassandra, and Kelly Ann all sob loudly.)

So, I leave to be divided among the three of you, and your families, the amount of *one dollar*.

(The daughters interrupt their crying and stand quickly.)
Kathleen, Cassandra, Kelly Ann: One dollar?

Gwen: Yes, that's right. One dollar. Now sit down.

(They sit.)

I know you are surprised, but you shouldn't be. Family, I meant what I said. I love all of you tremendously, and all of you . . . love my money. I have always given each of you what you want out of life, and now I am going to try and give you what you need. And what you all need is a change of heart. You are all heartless and selfish. You love two things only—money and yourselves. That's not what life is about. You want to know what life is about? Ask Ben—he knows. He's had to go without food and family before, and now he is thankful to God that he has them both. I wish all of you were that way, and I know you can be. In fact, I am so sure you can change that I am going to ask you to do just that. I am going to ask each of you to change specific things, and if after one year, you have successfully done so, you will receive a great reward. Your reward will be a happier life. However, I know all of you well enough to realize that that alone is not incentive enough. So, if you are *all* successful, you will get all my money back after one year.

All: What?!

Gwen: Kathleen, I want you to be the loving person I know you can be. Put a smile on that face! Tell your girls you love them, but mostly, show them. Be patient with them and lower your decibel level, you know, cut out the screaming. Cassandra, I want you to be appreciative. Appreciate Owen and Ben. They try so hard to please you. Don't be so persnickety! And stop worrying about having a baby. When the Lord wants you to have a baby you will have one, so put it out of your mind. Kelly Ann, I want you to get a job and get a husband.

Kelly Ann: What?

Gwen: Believe it or not, there *is* a man out there who is good enough for you, and if you don't shape up, you're going to lose him before you find him! You must be married one year from today, or else you'll be one very poor spinster. Now Marilyn, Rebecca, and Gracie—I have a word for you too. Change while you can. Learn now about what's really meaningful in life and your life will seem . . . more meaningful! Mind your manners—and your mother! Owen, please continue managing the lumber yard and let Ben help you. After all, he is the first grandson, so very soon Acklen Lumber Yard will be his. I have one last request for all of you. (more serious) For years now, I have risen every Sunday morning to a quiet household with bedroom doors shut tightly and everyone sleeping soundly. I have tiptoed around getting ready for church, afraid that if I made too much noise and awakened anyone, I'd get my head bitten off for ruining their "one day of the week they can sleep in." My children, Sundays are *not* meant for sleeping in. Sunday mornings are meant for rising early and rushing around trying to get ready for Sunday School and church. Remember, girls? Remember when you were little? Oh, how these quiet Sunday mornings have saddened me. Ben, I thank you for your company *every* Sunday morning. I thank you also for your commitment to God. I will also remind you three girls of your commitments to Him. I expect all of you to be present at church each Sunday from now on. This is the most vital requirement! Well, that's all I have to say. Please, do this—for me. I will miss all of you. But don't worry about me. I am safe and very happy. Good-bye, my children!

Kathleen: What does she mean by "safe and happy"?

Cassandra: Oh, it is obvious she's referring to her new heavenly life.

Kathleen: Lillian, why would our mother go away and not tell us she was ill? Is she dying? Is she afraid to burden us?

Lillian: Listen, everyone, safe and happy means just that . . . she is safe and happy. I wish I could tell you more but I cannot.

Kelly Ann: Well, perhaps you can tell me *why* she decided to withhold my inheritance. Hmm? Can you tell me that Miss Lillian Laraby, attorney at law?

Lillian: I think she made that clear to all of you. And she's only withholding your inheritances for a year, during which time I will make regular visits to see how you are progressing. In the meantime, who should I give this to? (presents a one-dollar bill)

Kelly Ann: Well, don't you have change?

Cassandra: Yes, do you want us to cut it into thirds?

Kathleen: (harshly) Gracie, go get 100 pennies from your piggy bank! (realizing she has screamed) Uh, I mean, Gracie Dear, would you please go get change from your piggy bank so we can divide this dollar?

(Gracie leaves.)

Cassandra: This is the most ridiculous thing I have ever heard of.

Kelly: How could mother do this to me? I have to be married in one year? And I have to do it on a budget of 33¢?

(Gracie re-enters and gives 100 pennies to Lillian who divides them three ways.)

Kathleen: No, Kelly Ann, you'll get a job, remember? All of us will; we'll all help out.

(Lillian has now distributed thirty-three pennies to each daughter. Then, they divide it among their families.)

Lillian: Well, that just about does it. Who gets the extra penny?

All: I do! I do!

Kathleen: (Once again they are reminded of their greediness.) Uh, what we meant, was, uh, why don't you keep it, Lillian Dear? After all, you've helped give us so much insight into ourselves.

Lillian: Well, I am not allowed to keep it. I'll leave it on the table, and you can decide who gets it. I'll be going now. You call me if you have any questions. Good-bye.

Owen: I'll see you out.

(There is a long pause, and they all sit stunned.)

Cassandra: What are we going to do? What ever are we going to do?

Kathleen: I think the three of us should divide up with our families and discuss this. We have a lot of changes to make, and frankly I'm still in shock. Come on, girls.

Owen: Kathleen, you are absolutely right. Ben, Cassandra, let's go upstairs.

(Kathleen, Marilyn, Rebecca, Gracie, Owen, Cassandra, and Ben exit.)

(Kelly Ann is left alone on stage, and she stands deserted with her hands on her hips. She finds comfort in counting her pennies for a while and then she speaks:)

Kelly Ann: Oh, this is unspeakable! What do I do, discuss it with myself? I don't have a family of my own to discuss this with. I don't want one either. One year. Oh, how can I be married in one year with such little money? (She strolls off counting her pennies, then stops abruptly and turns. She darts to the table where the extra penny has been left, and after snatching it, she exits happily.)

END OF ACT ONE

ACT TWO

It is four months later. The family's improvements are minor, but they are trying. Kathleen is hurrying to leave for a PTA meeting. Cassandra is going into town for a shopping spree and a doctor's appointment, and Kelly Ann has a job interview.

Scene One

Kathleen: (from offstage) Marilyn! Where are you? (She enters darning a sock that is on her foot.) Marilyn! Get down here! (she stops and realizes she has been yelling) Oh, Marilyn darling, would you please come here?

Marilyn: Yes, Mother?

Kathleen: Marilyn, where are my clean socks?

Marilyn: I don't know, Mother. Rebecca has laundry duty this week. Gracie and I are in charge of housework. (enter Cassandra)

Kathleen: I am never going to get to that PTA meeting on time. Cassandra, are you going?

Cassandra: No, Kathleen. I am not a teacher.

Kathleen: Yes, but you are a parent, and without parents there would be no "P" in "PTA."

Cassandra: Well, I simply can't go. I am going shopping this morning and then I am going for my annual physical at Doc Curtis'.

(enter Gracie cleaning and Rebecca with laundry)
(also enter Kelly Ann)

Kelly Ann: Good morning, all! Oh, Rebecca! Thank you for washing my dress, dear, and now, I must iron it.

Kathleen: Well, well, well, good morning, Miss Sunshine. Did you put too much sugar in your coffee or did you go out with Lesley again last night?

Kelly Ann: Now, now, it isn't either of those. Well, things have been going well with Lesley, but you know, he is so poor. And besides, he has never given me that lavender piano he promised me. No, prepare yourselves. I have a job interview today!

Cassandra: Well, it's about time. It's been four months since you were told to get a job.

Kelly Ann: (walks away and leaves iron on dress)
Well, I am going to be a secretary, I think. Yes, I think I can do that. After all, I am very polite on the telephone. (turns back to dress) Oh no! My dress!

(enter, Ben and Owen)

Kelly Ann: Owen, you're just in time. Fix that nasty iron. It has ruined my dress!

Kathleen: Ben, make yourself useful over there and help me look for a good pair of socks.

Cassandra: Hey, everyone, don't yell at my men! Good morning, Ben, good morning, Owen.

Owen: Good morning, Dear.

Kathleen: (yelling) I did not yell. I don't yell anymore.

(Entire family begins to bicker and the doorbell rings.)

Scene Two

Kelly Ann: I'll get it. (She answers door, still in her robe, to find Pastor Foster and his family there. She slams the door and screams.)

Kathleen: Kelly Ann, who is it?

Kelly: It's *Pastor Frazier!*

(Everyone scurries to tidy up the house and themselves.)

Ben: His name is Pastor Foster, Aunt Kelly.

Kathleen: Oh, Pastor Foster—My, oh my, what a breeze there is today! (She fans the door.) Please come in!

(enter the Fosters—all smiling)

Wilson: Good morning to all of you! Good morning, Ben! I hope this isn't a bad time?

Owen: Oh no, come in, Sir, this is as good a time as any. (laughs nervously)

Wilson: I've seen you at church a few times since your mother's unfortunate departure. But, I have never had the opportunity to introduce my family to your family. This is my wife, Miriam, our youngest daughter, little Liza. This is Sara Beth, and this is our son, Cory.

(Marilyn, Rebecca, and Gracie all sigh and giggle—then Rebecca is shoved toward Cory.)

Miriam: Oh, I am so pleased to meet you. Gwendolyn has told me so much about each of you that I feel as if I know you. Hello, which daughter are you? (they shake hands) Oh no, wait, you must be Kelly Ann. Gwendolyn told me you weren't married (points to empty ring finger on left hand).

Kelly: Yes, well, it seems that mother has alerted the media about that. Excuse me, I have an appointment, and I really must get dressed.

Miriam: It was nice to meet you! Now, you must be Cassandra and Owen, Ben's parents. Ben has been so helpful to us at the church. He is a real example to the other youth at church.

Cassandra and Owen: He is?

Miriam: That leaves Kathleen, and that must be you. I'm Miriam, and I want you to know that I admire you for raising three children all alone. I could never manage it. How do you do it?

Kathleen: Uh, well, I just take it one day at a time. (Cassandra lets out a *ha!* Kathleen shoves her just as Miriam turns to them so they smile sweetly.)

Miriam: Well, you must be the Acklen granddaughters. Now then, which one of you is Rebecca?

(The girls giggle.)

Rebecca: (nervously) I am Pastor Foster. I mean, Mrs. Pastor Foster, I mean Mrs. Foster. (pauses, then sighs) Hi, Cory.

Cory: Hello, Rebecca. You look very nice this morning.

(The girls sigh and giggle.)

Rebecca: Thank you, Cory. You look very tall, I *mean*, I *mean*, you look very nice . . . too. That's what I meant. You look very nice.

Wilson: I am sorry we have delayed this visit, but, well, you were coming regularly for a while. We haven't seen you lately.

Cassandra: Pastor Foster, you're right. We haven't been lately, and mother would have wanted us to. I am afraid we have failed her miserably.

Wilson: Well, now, our church's door is always open. We'd love to have all of you at our church, but if you wish to attend elsewhere that's fine. The most important thing is that you all get involved *somewhere*.

Kathleen: Pastor, it's only fair that we tell you that we haven't been attending anywhere. And we shouldn't either. We three girls were raised and baptized there. Our memberships are still at First Baptist, Gibsonville, and that's where we should go. What do you think, Gang?

All: Yes, you're right.

Miriam: Oh, good, that's wonderful! Ladies, I'd love to have you all at our Ladies' Bible Study this Thursday morning. It's at the church at 9:30.

Wilson: Yes, and Owen, we are trying to add a new playground facility for the children at the church, and I'd like to discuss some prices with you on your lumber. (starts to leave)

Owen: Why, of course we will! We can donate as much as you need! Everyone, let's see the Fosters to their car. (They all exit except Cory and Rebecca.)

Cory: Hi again.

Rebecca: Hi!

Cory: I've missed seeing you at church. Why have you stopped coming?

Rebecca: I didn't want to stop coming. I'm not old enough to drive yet, and my family quit going. I have wanted to come.

Cory: Well, I'm old enough to drive. Do you think your mother would allow me to pick you up on Sundays?

Rebecca: (stares and smiles) Oh, Cory, that is so sweet! Oh, but if I do that, my mom will have no incentive to get up and go herself. I'd better go with my family.

Cory: Now *that's* really thoughtful. Are you always so thoughtful?

Rebecca: (eagerly) Oh yes! I am always thoughtful—why, I think all the time!!!

Cory: Rebecca?

Rebecca: (quickly, almost overlapping him) Yes?

Cory: Would you spend some time thinking about accompanying me to the Youth Spring Supper next month?

Rebecca: Next month? How can you be sure that you will still want to go with me next month?

Cory: I'm just sure, that's all. But if you don't want to go . . .

Rebecca: No! I mean, yes, I do. Of course, I do. I'd love to. (They sigh deeply.)

Cory: Well, I'd better go before my folks leave me.

(Lesley appears at the open front door and is confused as to whether he should walk in or knock.)

Scene Three

Lesley: Excuse me. Uh, hello? (Cory and Rebecca jump up from where they are seated.)

Rebecca: Hello, may I help you?

Lesley: Yes. Yes, is Kelly Ann at home?

Rebecca: Sure. Aunt Kelly Ann, there is someone here to see you.

Kelly Ann: (from offstage) Who is it?

Rebecca: (to Lesley) Who is it?

Rebecca: Tell her Lesley is here.

Rebecca: It's Lesley.

Kelly Ann: Oh! OK.

Rebecca: Good-bye, Cory. I enjoyed our talk.

Cory: Good-bye, Becca.

(Rebecca walks him to the door and then turns to Lesley.)

Rebecca: So, are you the lucky guy?

Lesley: Excuse me?

Rebecca: Are you going to marry my Aunt Kelly Ann?

Lesley: Well, well, uh, what's your name?

Rebecca: Rebecca.

Lesley: Well, Rebecca, I don't quite know what our long-range plans are, but our immediate plans are just to enjoy each other's company.

Rebecca: Well, don't enjoy each other's company for too long. My Aunt Kelly Ann has only eight more months and then... (makes a cutting motion at the neck)

Lesley: What? Is she sick of something?

Rebecca: No! If she doesn't marry somebody in eight months, she will be disinherited. She's gone out with you a few times, so I just thought you were the lucky fellow!

Lesley: Oh no. I didn't know about the inheritance deadline.

(enter Kelly Ann)

Kelly Ann: Hello, Mr. Piano Man. Good-bye, Rebecca.

(Rebecca exits)

Lesley: Hello, Kelly Ann.

Kelly Ann: Aren't you going to tell me how beautiful I look? I have an engagement!

Lesley: An engagement? To whom?

Kelly Ann: No, no, silly. An appointment. Are you feeling OK?

Lesley: Yes. Kelly Ann, are you marrying me for the money?

Kelly Ann: Ha! My weekly allowance is more than your monthly salary. Or, well, it used to be. No, I am not marrying you for the money!

Lesley: Of course, I meant, you are *planning* on marrying me for your money? You see, I heard about your eight-month deadline.

(changing the subject) Have you located a lavender piano yet?

Lesley: Please don't change the subject.

Kelly Ann: Oh, all right. No, I am not using you to get my inheritance—yet. I don't even know if I like you. (long pause) Oh, all right, I like you. Are you happy?

Lesley: Yes, very.

Kelly Ann: Well, good because I am late.

Lesley: Kelly Ann, can I see you tonight?

Kelly Ann: Well, yes, I suppose you can. In fact, I suppose I would like that. I will be ready by, I mean, when would you like me to be ready, Lesley?

Lesley: At 7?

Kelly Ann: That's great! What would you like to do?

Lesley: What?

Kelly Ann: What would you like to do?

Lesley: Kelly Ann, that's the first time you have ever asked me what *I'd* like to do.

Kelly Ann: Is it?

Lesley: Yes (tenderly) and thank you. (He kisses her on the cheek.)

Kelly Ann: (in disbelief after a long pause) You're welcome, Lesley. I'll see you tonight.

Lesley: Are you leaving now for your appointment?

Kelly Ann: What? Oh, yes! Shall we leave together?

Lesley: Certainly.

(They leave and the stage is bare for a few seconds. Cassandra enters dazed, carrying several shopping bags. She sits at the table by a pitcher of water. Marilyn and Gracie come bursting in from outside.)

Scene Four

Cassandra: Girls, where is your Uncle Owen?

Marilyn: He's been outside talking with Pastor Foster most of the day.

Cassandra: Oh. That's nice. (still dazed) Would you please get him for me?

(they leave, and she reaches in her purse)

Cassandra: Oh, I need an Excedrin. No, maybe I shouldn't.

Owen: Hello, Cassie, you look so vibrant this morning. Have you been out shopping?

Cassandra: Yes, Owen.

Owen: Well, you must have found a new toy for yourself. Did you find something you like?

Cassandra: Yes, Owen.

Owen: Well . . . am I ever going to see it?

Cassandra: Yes, Owen.

Owen: When?

Cassandra: Well (long pause), you'll see it in October, Owen.

Owen: (still wondering) What could possibly have to wait until (Slowly he turns as if he has understood.) *October, Owen?* Cassie, are we, am I, are you finally . . . ?

Cassandra: (finally excited) Yes, Owen!

Owen: (shouting) Are you positive?

Cassandra: I am positive. It is positive. You are positive! We are all positive!

Owen: Oh, Cassandra, things have been so good between us lately, and this just tops everything. Let's go tell the others! Come on! (He helps her up.) Be careful now!

Scene Five

(Seven months have passed now, and the lights come up on an empty house. The phone begins to ring. Enter Kelly Ann and Lesley from upstairs.)

Kelly Ann: Hello? Oh, hello, Miss Lillian Laraby, attorney at law, how are you today? (pause) Yes, I know it is time for one of your visits again, but I am afraid that not everyone is here. If I plan this month's visit without considering everyone else's schedule they might not be here when you come to observe our behavior. How much longer will we be under your surveillance? (pause) Two months? Well, I suppose the worst is behind us. Why don't you stop by tonight? I'll tell everyone to be present. Good-bye.

Lesley: See there, you *can* be polite.

Kelly Ann: Yes, and it didn't even hurt!

Lesley: Did I hear you say you have two months longer to be under surveillance?

Kelly Ann: Yes, why?

Lesley: Does that mean you have two more months to meet your marriage deadline? (takes out a pocket calendar)

Kelly Ann: Why, yes, it's two months from today, Friday, November 24, 1988. I'll never forget that dreadful morning we all heard that ugly video will!

Lesley: So, you must be married by November 24th of this year, 1989?

Kelly Ann: Yes, it's a Saturday, I believe.

Lesley: Yes, it is, are you busy that day?

Kelly Ann: I don't know if I'll be busy or what. That's two months from now. Why?

Lesley: Kelly Ann, we have been dating for ten months now.

Kelly Ann: Yes, I know. I have been waiting that long for my lavender piano.

Lesley: Is that the only reason you've been seeing me?

Kelly Ann: (long pause) No, it isn't.

Lesley: Kelly Ann, I am not rich enough to buy you a big ring, or even a purple piano.

Kelly Ann: Lavender.

Lesley: Yes, well, I am not rich, but I am smart. I am smart enough not to let you slip away from me. Not now and not ever. I think I can always make you happy. Now I'm not asking you this just to meet that deadline; it's just that, I have known for a long time.

Kelly Ann: Known what?

Lesley: Kelly Ann Acklen, I want you to be my wife. (pulls out a small box and Kelly Ann begins to open it. It contains a small, lavender piano music box.)

Kelly Ann: It's my purple piano!

Lesley: Lavender. I looked everywhere for lavender.

Kelly Ann: Oh yes, lavender. It's wonderful, and Lesley, so are you. Only . . .

Lesley: What?

Kelly Ann: Well, I cannot marry you.

Lesley: Why not?

Kelly Ann: Well, two months is just not enough time to plan a formal wedding. And besides, if I marry you I'll be... (pause) KELLY ANN KELLY!! Oh! Even worse, the government might delete my middle name and I would be KELLY KELLY!!

Lesley: Yes, I have thought about that. But I don't care, Kelly Ann. I want to marry you. I'll beg you.

Kelly Ann: Oh, please do.

Lesley: Please do me the honor of being my wife.

Kelly Ann: (There is a long pause, and then she turns to him.) Oh yes, yes, I will! I don't care if I will be a Kelly Kelly. I'll be the happiest Kelly Kelly that ever lived. Yes! I *will* marry you!

Lesley: Well, now you are busy on Saturday, November 24th!

Kelly Ann: No. Lesley, let's get married the next day, Sunday the 25th.

Lesley: But then you won't receive your inheritance. That's too late.

Kelly Ann: I don't care. I've always dreamed of a Sunday wedding.

Lesley: You mean, you would give up your inheritance just to have an ideal wedding with me?

Kelly Ann: Yes, I would. Mother is right. Money can't bring happiness. Only love can. Oh, Lesley, I am happy too. I am finally happy. Oh, I have so much planning to do! I am so excited I think I could shout at the top of my lungs!

(offstage Cassandra screams)

Lesley: What was that?

Kelly Ann: Oh, it sounded like Cassandra. Oh, Lesley, when she finds out I'm to be married, she'll probably go right into labor!

Kelly Ann and Lesley: Cassandra!

(Kathleen and Cassandra enter.)

Kathleen: Lesley, call that number by the phone and tell the doctor that Cassandra's water has broken.

Kelly Ann: Oh, Cassandra, is it time?

Cassandra: Oh, yes, oh, this is so exciting! Oh... this is so *painful!*

Kathleen: Oh, Cassandra you aren't really in labor yet. You'll be fine, Dear. Owen is coming with the suitcase, and you'll be on your way. Do you need anything?

Cassandra: Yes.

Kelly Ann and Kathleen: What?

Cassandra: (seriously yet still in pain) I need some courage. I'm scared. I've waited so many years to experience this, and now I don't think I can go through with it.

Kelly Ann: Well, Cassandra, I don't think you have much choice at this stage of the development.

Cassandra: Oh, Kelly Ann, you couldn't possibly understand!

Kelly Ann: Well, I might very soon!

Cassandra and Kathleen: What?

Kelly Ann: Oh no, not that! But I am going to be married. Lesley just asked me, and I have accepted. (Lesley joins them.)

Cassandra and Kathleen: This is wonderful, Kelly Ann! (They congratulate her and are interrupted by her labor pain.)

Cassandra: Oh!

Lesley: The doctor said to meet him at the hospital.

Cassandra: Oh, I'm still so scared. What can I do?

Kathleen: Well, why don't we do what Mother would do if she were here?

Cassandra: (pause) Yes, let's.

(Circled around Cassandra, they all bow their heads and pray silently. The lights fade.)

Scene Six

(It is one month later, Thanksgiving Day, 1989. Gwendolyn enters with a suitcase.)

Gwen: Well, they haven't changed the locks. (looking around) Hello, home. (walks to mantel) Hello, Wendall. (whispering still) Happy Thanksgiving, everyone. At least, I hope this will be a happy Thanksgiving. Goodness knows, last Thanksgiving was a disaster. A lot can happen in a year, and I have sure missed my family. I am very anxious to see if . . . (She is interrupted by the sound of Kathleen's voice and she hides.)

Kathleen: Come and see, everyone! Come and see the beautiful Thanksgiving turkey Owen has carved!

Lesley: Yes, Owen, the turkey looks wonderful. However, would it be possible for me to carve the turkey next year?

Owen: Why, sure! It's easy as pie.

Ben: Speaking of pie, is the pie ready, Mother?

Cassandra: Yes, Honey. Marilyn is bringing it. Little Wendall is enough of a handful. I couldn't manage the pie and the baby, so I brought what was most important. Isn't that right, Wendall? You are much more important than some silly old pie, aren't you? Would the baby like some pumpkin pie?

Kathleen: (lovingly) Come on, Girls. We're waiting on you.

Gracie: Well, here we all are!

Rebecca: Yes, and there's two more at the table this year, Baby Wendall and Lesley.

Marilyn: On Sunday, that will be *Uncle Lesley.*

Kathleen: Well, there may be two more of us, but there is still someone missing. I think we all miss her very much. You know, we should all take turns telling something we are thankful for. Then, after that, we can thank God for this year's blessings and then eat.

(They do so. Starting with Gracie and going around to Cassandra. Since a real change needs to be seen in the characters here, the cast is requested to improvise this section, to make it seem genuine. After Cassandra finishes she adds:)

Cassandra: I am most thankful for this little cherub—uh oh, this little cherub seems to have soaked his diaper. I just changed him; that was fast! (she rises) Owen, go ahead and bless the food, and I'll be right back.

Owen: Dear Lord, thank you for such a wonderful Thanksgiving Day. But Lord, thank You the most for such a good year. Thank You for all the hard times that made it so wonderful . . . eventually. We know now that You just want us to seek You. Thank You for this food. In Jesus' name I pray, Amen!

(While they have been praying, Gwen has come to the head of the table. They open their eyes and scream loudly.)

Kathleen: Mother!

Everyone: Mother/Grandmother (They jump up and run to her.)

Kelly Ann: Mother! Where have you been and why are you back? Oh,

Mother, we thought you were gone forever!

Kathleen: Mother, we've missed you. It's been a terribly hard year without you, hasn't it, Girls?

Girls: Yes, it has!

Gwen: Well, it looks like the year hasn't been too terrible. Look at all of you! You look wonderful, and you look happy!

Marilyn: Oh, we are, Grandmother!

Ben: Yes, especially now that you're home.

Kelly Ann: Mother, why did you leave? Is it why I think?

Gwen: Why do you think I left?

Kelly Ann: Because some people don't know what they've got until it's gone!

Kathleen: Yes, and you left to help us to see that, didn't you?

Gracie: Grandmother, we do know, all of us, how fortunate we are, especially to have you back home.

Kelly Ann: Yes, but most of all, we are all happy, Mother. Really happy. And . . . we're poor! Speaking of poor, Mother, meet your future son-in-law, Lesley Kelly.

Gwen: None of you are poor anymore. You have earned your inheritances in a way, because I am back! Now, Lesley, I have heard a lot about you!

Kathleen: From whom? Where have you been?

Gwen: I have been with Lillian.

Kelly Ann: You mean Lillian Laraby, attorney at law?

Gwen: Yes. She has kept me abreast of everything.

Owen: I don't know why we didn't figure that out. She was over here once a month like clockwork. By chance, did she tell you any other news?

Gwen: Yes, she told me that Kathleen and the girls we're getting along beautifully, and that you and Cassandra were happier than ever.

Owen: Did she tell you why?

Gwen: No, Why?

(Cassandra starts to enter, and they all cover Gwen's eyes. Cassandra enters and sees her mother. She is surprised, yet very quiet. She stands proud of her son, almost tearful.)

Cassandra: Happy Thanksgiving, Mother.

Gwen: Cassandra! What? Lillian never told me about this. Who is this?

Cassandra: This is your grandson, Wendall Owen Beacham. We call him Wendall, after Daddy.

(For a very long while, everyone is quiet. Slowly they all mingle with each other, exchanging hugs and kisses during a quiet time of thanksgiving.)

Gracie: Well (drying her eyes), are we going to eat, or what? I am famished!

Gwen: Gracie, you said that last year! Oh honestly, I think I need to stand right here in this very spot and get an eyeful of all of you.

Kathleen: No, Mother. I think we owe you the Thanksgiving dinner you never received last year.

Cassandra: Yes. Come and sit down. Mother, why don't you bless the food again for us?

Gwen: I'd be happy to.

(They all bow their heads and close their eyes. Gwen keeps her eyes open and stares at each family member briefly. Then she looks toward heaven and mouths with no voice, "thank you," and winks. Then, she begins to sing "We Gather Together." Everyone looks up and joins in with her to complete the verse, after which they all clap, and then share their very first *thankful* Thanksgiving dinner.)

(lights fade to closing music.)

THE END

THE HEALING

by
Laura Harris Smith

SYNOPSIS - THE HEALING

Emmett Lee Westbrook is a well educated, celebrated author and father of three children who buries himself in his work. Dorothy "Dory" Oakes is a much simpler woman, who at the age of 56 has never been married.

So why have Emmett and Dory been together for 20 years? Because Dorothy is the Westbrooks' nanny and housekeeper and has devoted her life to them since the death of Mrs. Grace Westbrook, who died 21 years before of a genetic disorder called Huntington's Disease. Now with the children raised and gone, Dorothy remains to care for Mr. Westbrook, which is no easy job! All work and no play has made Emmett Westbrook a difficult and demanding father, who sadly, is visited by his children only on spasmodic holidays. Even this is arranged by Dory, since Emmett never contacts the children. With the use of a scrim and an alternate stage, *The Healing*'s audience is repeatedly transported back in time to view a much different Westbrook family before the death of their mother.

The play begins as Dory schemes to invite all the children home for Christmas despite the fact that she knows this will unhinge Emmett. Millie, the oldest, is a successful editor for a St. Louis newspaper, and is married and expecting her first baby. Ethan, Emmett's only son, is unmarried, uninspired and yet his carefree spirit is refreshing in comparison to his "all work" father. Of course, Emmett is not pleased with this display of irresponsibility and Ethan and Millie have both stayed away for nine months. Annie, Emmett's youngest daughter, has not been home in five years. Although she once was the apple of his eye (as we see in the powerful "flashback" scenes) because of a disapproved marriage, she has stayed away at Emmett's request. Now at 25, she finds herself drained, unhealthy and abandoned by her husband. She has the added pressure of raising her 5-year-old daughter, Emma, all alone. Nonetheless, Dory arranges the reunion and eagerly prepares for their homecoming.

Separately, the children arrive in Brookport, Illinois. Accompanying Annie and Emma is Claudia Carney, Emmett's flamboyant 1st cousin, who has known some success as a Broadway actress and provides comic relief to tension at the Westbrook home. Emmett, who won't budge an inch, continues to neglect his children, especially when he learns that his granddaughter, Emma, is deaf. As family communication reaches its worst, Dory finally decides to give Emmett a piece of her mind, and she divertingly ties him to a chair to do so. Just when it seems Emmett might be ready for a reconciliation with Annie, Ethan decides that his sister's ill-health is too mysterious and needs investigating. In a gripping scene, Ethan discovers that Annie displays the fatal symptoms of HD, their family's genetic disorder, and he and Millie pray for a healing. Their prayers for a healing are soon answered, but not as they expected. In a tense, yet memorable moment surrounding Annie's impending death, Emmett and Annie receive the emotional healing they need, and through Emma, Emmett is given the added blessing of a second chance at fatherhood.

The Healing is a poignant drama dealing with the delicate subjects of death, estranged families and the handicapped child, while also revealing the painful consequences that neglect and divorce can bring to a family. Moreover, *The Healing* is a moving testimony of one family's miracle, with the added reminder that to limit God is to deprive ourselves of the higher healing that rests just within our reach.

SETTING

The play is set in Brookport, Illinois, population 1,128. It is Christmastime, 1989. The entire play takes place from Friday, December 22, to Monday, December 25, in the home of Emmett Lee Westbrook. It is a beautiful home in Brookport, resting just on the Illinois/Kentucky border.

CHARACTERS

Emmett Lee Westbrook—A celebrated author and father of three children. He is a stern, stoic man and has buried himself in his work since the death of his wife in late 1968. He is 54 years old, attractive, and well-groomed.

Dorothy Oakes—From Paducah, Kentucky, Dorothy is a delightful, humorous, but bossy Southern nanny. She came to work as the Westbrook's housekeeper and nanny in 1969 and remains there to care for Mr. Westbrook, even though all his children are now grown. Dorothy never had a family of her own and has devoted her entire life to the Westbrooks. She is 56 years old.

Millicent Kae Adams—Known to the family as "Millie," she is the oldest of Emmett's children. She is 30 years old and lives in Saint Louis, Missouri, with her husband Kurt. She is well educated yet very humble. She works for a St. Louis newspaper.

Ethan Westbrook—Ethan is 26 and the middle child. He also resides in St. Louis, moving there after he dropped out of college several years before. He is not wealthy but is still happy and carefree nonetheless. He is gentle, compassionate, tall, and attractive.

Charlotte Ann Scott—25, and the youngest of the Westbrook children, she is affectionately referred to as "Annie" by everyone except her father. Her name means "small, womanly, and full of grace" and she exemplifies this perfectly. After marrying Jeffrey Scott against her father's wishes, they moved to New York where they later had a baby girl, Emma. She has not been home in five years, and only her sister has seen Emma.

Claudia Carney—The same age as Emmett her first cousin, she is very youthful for her age. She also lives in New York and has remained in close contact with Annie. She has known some success as an actress, both on and off-Broadway. She has never married, but claims to have several boyfriends. She is tall and slender, also flamboyant, pretentious, and swanky.

Emma Lee Scott—Annie's only child, Emma is five years old. She is well-behaved and cute, but she has been deaf since birth.

Dr. Martin Grayson—Also from Brookport, he is a long-time friend of the Westbrooks. He was the doctor who treated Grace Westbrook when she was ill. He is 51 years old.

Grace Ann Westbrook—Although she has been dead for 21 years, we are able to see her through her family's remembrances. She is tall, dark, and elegantly beautiful. She epitomizes the perfect mother, being both patient and loving. After being stricken at an early age with Huntington's Disease, she died of pneumonia at age 32.

Young Emmett Westbrook—At this stage in his life he is a different man than the older Emmett. He is witty, loving, and a devoted family man. He is in his early 30's.

Young Claudia Carney—Even at 12 years of age she is exactly the same as she appears in adulthood.

Young Grace Ann—Although she and young Claudia appear in only one scene, in that scene that we learn about the beginning stages of her crippling disease. She is 10 years old in this crucial scene.

Young Millicent, Ethan, and Annie Westbrook.

ACT ONE

Scene One

(The lights come up on an empty stage. The phone rings, and Emmett yells from offstage.)

Emmett: Dorothy? Dorothy, get the telephone. (Emmett enters and answers phone) Westbrook. Yes, Lyndon. What did the publisher say? Excellent. Excellent. And when is the pub date? And they promise no delays this time? Good. Oh, did you eliminate the book-signing tour from the contract? What? Lyndon, I specifically requested that be changed.

There's no way I can write two more books in the next year if I'm spending every night in a different city socializing in a library. That just isn't me, Lyndon. Now see what you can do, OK? Tomorrow? Well, I guess I can. Can't my signature wait 'til after Christmas? Well, I'll see if I can fly in tomorrow or maybe Sunday. What? No, I haven't decided yet on the dedication page, but I will soon. I'll think about it on the plane and let you know. Thanks for the hard work, Lyndon. (Dory enters as he is hanging up.)

Dory: Sorry, Sir. I was running the vacuum and didn't hear the phone ring. That old vacuum is as dilapidated as I am. (aside) And as noisy, I suppose.

Emmett: Dorothy, I have good news.

Dory: I can buy a new vacuum?

Emmett: You can buy ten new vacuums. My new book is on the way to the printers.

Dory: Oh, Sir, how wonderful! Was that Mr. Peters on the phone?

Emmett: Yes, quite a Christmas gift, eh?

Dory: Yes Sir, it is, it is indeed. Hey! I know what—we'll celebrate. I'll thaw my biggest ham. Then, I'll go to the market and buy enough food to make all your favorite fixin's. And I'll bake some good dinner rolls too, but this time I'll leave off the poppy seeds, seein' as how they get lodged in your teeth now and then.

Emmett: Thank you, Dory.

Dory: Oh, Mr. Westbrook, I was wonderin'. Since I'm fixin' all this food, wouldn't it be fine if I . . . invited the children? (There is a long pause.) Well?

Emmett: I'm going into the office now. I'll call you with my decision.

Dory: No can do.

Emmett: And why not?

Dory: Because St. Louis is two hours away, and you'll wait around and call me at dinner time, and say, "Sure, Dorothy, invite them." Then it'll be too late for them to make the drive. Besides, it's three days before Christmas, and you got no business goin' to the office. And that's another thing— you've got this whole house to yourself, and yet you insist on going somewhere else to do your thinking. It's a waste of money, I say, a waste of money. I do all my writing at the kitchen table, and you could do the same. (He glances at the table to find it stacked with various items.)

Emmett: Dorothy, the only writing you do is to your Aunt Gladys.

Dory: I beg your pardon. If it were not for *me* writing to *your* children you'd never know anything about them! Sir, please. It's Christmas. May I call them?

Emmett: (After a pause he puts on his coat and gloves.) If you must. (starts to leave)

Dory: Oh, wait, you never read yesterday's mail. (hands it to him)

Emmett: Thank you.

Dory: Not much really, just *The Times, The Tribune, The Post,* and a donation request for the Huntington's Disease Society of America.

Emmett: Just give me the papers. (turns) Dory, how do you know this is a donation request?

Dory: I took the liberty and peeked.

Emmett: (sees that envelope is opened) Funny, I was under the impression that a person's mail was private.

Dory: Well, if you're not going to donate to the society, I am. Honestly, those good people are just trying to find a cure for HD. If more people had donated in the past perhaps *Mrs.* Westbrook would still be with you today.

Emmett: And if she were, Dorothy, you'd be out of a job.

Dory: Well, Sir, you do have a way with words. We'll discuss it later. (puts a scarf on him) Now, I'm gonna go get my address book and call the children. Have a good day. I hope you write a #1 best-seller! Bye now. (She exits.)

(Emmett slowly walks toward the door and stops. The stage lights fade and come up on a separate area with a spotlight. Enter a young Mrs. Westbrook with an ironing board and some pants.)

Grace: Millicent, Ethan, Annie, tell Father good-bye. He's leaving for work soon. (Enter young Mr. Westbrook dressed completely for work with shirt, tie, suitcoat, socks, shoes, hat, briefcase, but no pants. Just boxer shorts will do. Laughing, the children enter and gather around him.)

All children: Daddy! Daddy!

Young Emmett: Yes? Is there a problem, Millicent?

Millie: Daddy you're not dressed! (The children are laughing hysterically while Grace irons.)

Emmett: Well, let's see, do I have my shirt and tie?

Children: Yes! (laughing)

Emmett: Hmmm. Do I have my shoes and socks?

Children: Yes!

Emmett: Well, the last time I checked I had on my hat and coat, so I'll be on my way now. Bye.

Children: No, Daddy! Wait, you've lost something!

Emmett: Grace, do I appear to have lost something?

Grace: Yes, Dear—*your mind* (hands him the pants) . . . and your pants. You'd better hurry. Have a good day. (She adjusts his hat.) I hope you write a #1 best-seller! (They exit and the spot fades, with lights coming back up on mainstage. Emmett is still standing in the doorway and he comes back in to get his hat. Dory enters with book.)

Dory: Did you forget something?

Emmett: Only my pants . . . er, I mean, (pause) my hat. (He exits.)

Scene Two

(Dorothy picks up the phone and dials.) 1-212-293-6056. Yes, Claudia, it's Dory. I'm not used to speakin' into one of these things, but I was just callin' to see if you made your flight arrangements yet. I spoke with Emmett, and he said the kids could come for Christmas. It's a good thing seein' as how I'd already invited them! Hello? Hello? (hangs up phone) Nobody ever told me I was on the clock. If that don't beat all. Those decoder phones will answer a caller and hang up on them too. No tellin' what they'll be able to do next (Phone rings and she looks at it strangely. Hesitantly, she answers the phone.) Hello? Oh, Claudia! I just talked to your decoder phone. Where are you? At the airport? Fantastic! Yes, it worked! No, he didn't specifically say that Annie could come. But then, with her livin' in New York he probably didn't figure I meant to invite her at the last minute too. We'll just shock him. Well then, he can just fire me. Hey, did you do your part? She is? Oh, do let me say hello! Hello? (rapidly) Oh, glory be! Is this really my little Charlotte Ann? Annie, how are you? Oh, Baby, I can't believe you're comin' home to see me. I just can't believe it! 'Course, I should believe it seein' as how I been prayin' so hard for the last five years. Yes sir, five years I've been prayin' for you to bring that baby and sit her right down on my knee. How are you? (pause) Oh, I just know you've been so lonely after that Jeffrey Scott up and left you. Now Annie, I told you never to trust a man with two first names. Didn't I tell you that? It's a good thing I never met that boy, or I'd have to look him up and whup him! Well, it's all over now, sugar, and you and Emma are comin' home for Christmas! I can't believe it but I do! When does your flight arrive? Well, Millicent and Ethan left early this morning so they should be here soon. I'd better scoot to the market. Listen now, Baby, you fly safe and when you get on the plane you ask to meet the captain, you hear? And while he's shakin' your hand you look at his eyes and make sure they're not fuzzy. Oh, and give Emma some chewin' gum in case her ears stop up. Well, you be sweet now. I enjoyed our talk. Bye now! (hangs up phone) Merry Christmas, Dory! Ooh, if that don't do my heart good. Let's see now (checking grocery list) Potatoes, snaps, flour, tea bags. (Doorbell rings.) Dory, are you expectin' somebody this early? (Millicent steps in and sets a bag of groceries down.)

Millie: Dory? Hi, Dory!

Dory: Oh, Millie! Just look at you! Where's Ethan?

Millie: When he didn't see Daddy's car here, he dropped me off and went straight to his office to see him. How are you?

Dory: Oh, sassy as ever. Stand back now and let me look good at you. Oh, Millie Honey, you're so scrawny. Don't you eat? (gasps) Oh, Honey, did Kurt lose his job?

Millie: No, Dory. Oh, it's good to see you. And no, Kurt has not lost his job. In fact, he just found out this morning that he got the job I wrote to you about! That's why he's not here, but he should be driving up Monday for Christmas Day dinner.

Dory: Now listen to that! You've got two cars! You must be livin' high!

Millie: Oh, Dory!

Dory: Oh, Millie, you look so happy. Skinny but happy!

Millie: (stands) Dory, I can't be that skinny. I've gained five pounds. Can't you tell?

Dory: (looks) Five pounds? Where'd you put it?

Millie: (smiled secretly and pats her tummy)

Dory: What? Millie, are you and Kurt goin' to have a little baby?

Millie: Well, I hope it's little. Yes!

Dory: Oh, Merry Christmas! Oh, Honey, that is something! Wait here. (runs to refrigerator and pulls out a piece of chocolate cake)

Millie: What are you doing?

Dory: Here, Honey, eat up quick. You don't look like a mama.

Millie: Why not?

Dory: You ain't fluffy enough yet. But you will be after this weekend! I'm about to go to the market for tonight's dinner.

Millie: Oh, that reminds me (goes to get bag)—I went for you. I knew just what father would want, too. I bought all his favorites. (removes food from bag) Potatoes, snap beans, rolls . . .

Dory: Any poppy seeds?

Millie: No.

Dory: Perfect! Now I can sit and visit with you! Oh! Guess who is goin' to be sittin' right here at this very table tonight?

Millie: Let me see. Is cousin Claudia flying in from New York?

Dory: Yes, but that's not all.

Millie: Dory, did you convince Annie to come home?

Dory: No, I got Claudia to do it, seein' as how they're so close and all. She and Emma are coming!

Millie: Oh, it's a miracle, Dory!

Dory: Yes. Oh no!

Millie: What?

Dory: I don't have a thing in the house for a baby to eat!

Millie: Dory, Emma's not a baby. She's five now. Gosh, I guess I haven't seen her since she was just crawling. Annie has sent me lots of pictures, though. I can hardly wait. (fearfully) What did Daddy say?

Dory: Well . . .

Millie: Dory! You haven't told him! Oh boy, Daddy hates surprises.

Dory: Well, he shouldn't. He should be ashamed of himself forbiddin' her to come here with Jeff. Now, I didn't like what I heard about the boy either, but Annie did the right thing. She loyally defended her husband and honored her father's wishes by stayin' away. He can't be mad at her.

Millie: But he is! He's mad just because she married him, Dory.

Dory: Well, that problem no longer exists. Poor thing. We should give her a weekend she'll never forget. (enter Ethan)

Scene Three

Ethan: Knock, knock! Anybody home? Oh, I'm sorry. I've got the wrong house. (exits)

Dory: Ethan! Ethan Westbrook, you get yourself back in here. (They hug.) Oh, Ethan, look at you! You grew up good!

Ethan: Thank you, Dory. It's all that Kentucky cornbread you made me eat. Hey, Millie, have you let that cat outa the bag yet?

Millie: Oh, Ethan, do be more civil, please. Yes, she knows about the baby. Didn't you find Daddy at the office?

Ethan: No, I chickened out. I figured if he got me alone he'd drill me about how much money I'm making, and about how much more I'd be making if I had finished college. I decided to wait and see him here.

Millie: Where Dory can defend you.

Dory: Ethan, don't you be ashamed. You haven't been without a job since you dropped out of school and I'm proud of you. Here, peel potatoes.

Ethan: Thanks, Dory. I've missed you too!

Dory: Well, then, why haven't you been home since Easter? You too, Missy.

Millie: Dory, I wish I came home more. Honest I do. But this isn't home anymore. Oh it's the same house I grew up in, but I think I speak for Ethan too when I say, I just don't feel welcome here anymore.

Dory: This family beats all I've ever seen. Gettin' together only at Christmas and Easter, *which,* by the way, is the only time your father attends church.

Millie: Oh, Daddy.

Ethan: I just don't get it. I wish you could have known him before Mom died. They were both so involved down at Brookport Baptist. He never travelled—he was writing for the paper then, and he'd always be home by 5. And, boy, did he have a great sense of humor! Remember?

Millie: Yes, but he doesn't anymore. He's just not the same man, Ethan. You know, I hate to say this, but I'm glad Mother isn't here to see him like this.

Dory: All right, you two give him some credit, will you? He went through a terrible time when your mother died. He watched her change from an attractive, graceful woman who loved him, to an unsightly, clumsy woman who hardly knew him. Huntington's Disease stripped your mother of everything she was, and everything he was too. Haven't you ever wondered why he never remarried? A new wife would have been much more practical than hiring me. And there have been plenty of women who liked your father, or at least, liked his money. Your father still loves your mother very much, and I think he misses that companionship.

Millie: He has you, Dory.

Dory: Hee! Yes, he has me. He has me vacuum. He has me cook, and he has me clean up afterwards.

Ethan: Well, if he were all that starved for companionship why has he cut off all communication with the three of us? Don't we remind him of the good times with Mom? (There is a long pause.) Oh, I see. You know, maybe that's the real reason he told Annie to stay away. She is so much like Mom. Her gentle disposition, I mean.

Millie: Oh, Ethan, that's absurd! There is no good excuse for a person not to see their children. But you are right about Annie being like Mother. Daddy would have to be blind not to notice that.

Dory: I certainly wish I had known your mother. She sounds like a fine woman!

Ethan: I've yet to find one like her.

Dory: Oh! Then you have been lookin'!

Ethan: Dory, what would you say if I told you I've been dating the same girl for six months?

Dory: Well, you know the first thing I'd ask. Can she cook?

Ethan: I don't know yet. But you taught me so well she won't need to!

Dory: I'm teasin' you. Hey, pick up that pot of potatoes. I want to hear all about her. Millie, are you finished with those snaps?

Millie: Almost. I'm coming. (Ethan and Dory exit chatting. Millie cleans off the table and tidies up the kitchen, slowly as if in deep thought. As she walks to the door, she stops and turns back to the room and stares. Suddenly from behind her, enter young Mrs. Westbrook and Millie and Annie as children.)

Grace: Girls, it's time to pour. Get the cake pans. (She pours.) Daddy sure will be surprised. He's going to have a very happy birthday. All right, who wants to lick the spoon?

Both: I do! I do! Please, Mommy!

Millie: Mother, she licked it last time!

Annie: Did not!

Millie: Yes, you did, you always do.

Annie: Do not!

Millie: Yes, you do. Doesn't she, Mommy? (They now notice their mother who has calmly begun to finish the batter herself.)

Grace: Mmm. This batter is good if I do say so myself. Share? (The girls nod.) That's better! Millicent, I want you to carefully place these pans in the oven. (She knocks the empty batter dish over, and it falls to the floor. She gets a brief look of frustration on her face and seems eager to send the girls on their way.) Annie, you carry this one. But be careful, the oven will be very hot. Run along now. (She goes to the water pitcher, takes a pill from her pocket, and swallows it, trying to regain her posture. The young Millicent has reappeared in the doorway and is watching her.)

Millie: Mommy, are you OK?

Grace: Yes, sweety, I just seem to be extra clumsy today. Don't worry about me. Let's go set that buzzer! (They exit past the older Millie who is still standing in the doorway.)

Ethan: Millie? Are you coming with those snap beans?

Millie: (coming out of the daze) Yes. (takes a deep breath, grabs her bowl and exits)

Scene Four

(Lights come up on an empty stage. Enter Emmett from the front door. He comes in and removes his coat.)

Emmett: Dorothy?

(enter Ethan)

Ethan: Hello, Dad.

Emmett: Ethan! When did you get in? (They shake hands.)

Ethan: A few hours ago. I was going to come by the office but . . . I didn't! (laughs nervously) How was your day?

Emmett: Pretty quiet. (They sit.) I let Elizabeth go home early so she could get a head start on the holidays, and I had to review a contract I'm about to sign. My new book is being published under a new agreement, and I'm trying to work out some of the kinks.

Ethan: No major problems, I hope.

Emmett: No, I'm contracted to write two more books over the next year. That normally wouldn't be a problem. However, there seems to be a tour I can't get out of.

Ethan: A book signing tour?

Emmett: Yes, can you imagine?

Ethan: Sure! I wish someone would ask me for my autograph.

Emmett: Well, Son, that won't happen as long as you work for someone else.

(Ethan stands and there is a long pause.)

Emmett: Didn't your sister come with you?

Ethan: Sure did. In fact, she and Dory have been slaving over the stove preparing all your favorites. Act surprised, though.

(enter Millie)

Millie: Daddy!

Emmett: (cordially) Millicent. (They hug.) How are you?

Millie: I'm just fine, Daddy.

Emmett: And Kurt? Where is he?

Millicent: Well, he had some business to take care of, but he's driving up later. I've missed you—you look wonderful!

Emmett: Well, Dorothy takes good care of me.

Millie: Oh, Daddy, that reminds me. (begins setting table) This will be her twentieth Anniversary here with you, and I thought Christmas might be the perfect occasion to get her something special. You know, something to say thank you.

Emmett: Doesn't her paycheck do that?

Millie: Oh, Daddy, stop. I know you got her something.

Emmett: Yes, I doubled her Christmas bonus.

Millie: Daddy, you didn't!

Emmett: Yes, why?

Millie: Daddy (hesitantly), Dory has been here for twenty years. That's longer than me, Ethan, Annie, or even Mother lived here. Don't you ever give her anything besides money?

Emmett: Well, I have promised her a new vacuum cleaner.

Millie: Daddy!

Emmett: What!

Millie: Don't you think that's a little impersonal?

Ethan: Yeah, Dad. Can I have her bonus?

(enter Dory)

Millie: Oh! You two are inexcusable!

Scene Five

Dory: Well, isn't this a heartwarmin' vision? You're arguing just like old times! Dinner is ready now. (to Emmett) Behave yourself!

Millie: (quietly to Dory) Where are Annie and Cousin Claudia?

Dory: They're comin' but their plane was delayed. Your father likes dinner at 6 sharp, so we're goin' to have to start without them.

Millie: Oh, Dory, this looks wonderful, and I am ravenous!

Dory: Have you told your father the good news, Millie?

Emmett: No, she didn't. Did the *St. Louis Post* give you a promotion?

Millie: Well, no Sir. I didn't get a promotion.

Dory: Yes, she did! She's been promoted to the highest position she could have.

Ethan: Yeah, and Kurt helped.

Emmett: Kurt helped? I don't understand.

Millie: Ethan! Daddy, Kurt and I are having a baby. You're going to be a grandfather again. (There is no response.) Daddy, aren't you happy about that?

Emmett: Oh, of course. Yes, of course. I just . . . thought you were going to wait until you became more established at the *Post*.

Millie: Well, Daddy, that was eight months ago I said that, and I am more established now. I'm Lifestyles Editor. How much more established do you want me to be?

Dory: Let's pray. (bows her head)

Millie: (growing more angry) I'll be able to complete the majority of my work from my home several months after the baby comes.

Dory: I'm proud of you, honey. Let's pray. (bows her head)

Millie: (still looking at her father) I know you are, Dory. I could dig ditches and you'd be proud of me.

Dory: Let's pray now! Sir?

Emmett: (blandly) Dear God. Thank You for this food and bless it to the nourishment of our bodies. And uh, Lord, thank You for bringing Ethan and Millicent here safely. I know Millie and Kurt will make fine parents. Amen. (They pass the food.) Are you expecting twins?

Millie: What?

Emmett: Well, I just wondered why there are two extra plates set out tonight.

Dory: Well, sir, I was meaning to speak to you about that very thing.

(The doorbell rings)

Emmett: Who is that?

Millie: Ethan, why don't you get the door? Now!

(He opens the door and Annie stands alone. She and Ethan hug, and then Emmett sees her. He rises and stands in place, half-stunned, half angry. Everyone is watching Emmett.)

Annie: Hello, everyone. (pause) Merry Christmas.

Dory and Millie: Annie!

(Dory, who has begun to cry, moves toward her.)

Dory: I can't believe it. I told myself I wouldn't spill but I just can't help it, it's so good to see you! Gimme a hug, girl! You're so skinny!

Millie: Oh, Dory, you think everybody's too skinny. Hello, Annie. (They embrace happily.) Here, let me take your coat. Where's Claudia?

Annie: She's outside with Emma.

Millie: I cannot wait to see Emma!

Annie: There is something you all need to know. It's about Emma.

(enter Claudia and Emma)

Dory: There she is! There's my baby!

Ethan and Millie: Emma! (They rush to her.)

Claudia: Well, doesn't anyone care to say hello to moi?

Dory: Sorry, Claudia. (gives a quick hug) You're gonna have to excuse me. I've been waiting five years for this. (kneels) Come here youngin'!

(Emma runs and stands by her mother.)

Ethan: What's wrong, Emma, are you shy?

Millie: Don't let all these people frighten you, Honey. I'm your Aunt Millicent. Do you remember me?

Ethan: Never mind her. I'm Uncle Ethan. I'm the one who sent you the singing telegram for your birthday. Did you get it?

(There is a long pause.)

Annie: Emma didn't hear you, Ethan.

Ethan: I sent you the singing...

Annie: No, *Ethan*, she didn't hear any of you. Emma is deaf.

(After a long pause, Ethan, Millie and Dory all stand slowly.)

Millie: Why didn't you tell us, Annie?

Annie: I'm sorry. I am. I didn't want you to find out this way. I'm sorry if I've ruined everything.

Dory: Nonsense! You didn't do no such thing.

Ethan: How do we communicate with her?

Dory: We'll just hug and kiss her a lot!

Annie: She knows American sign language. But, of course, that doesn't help you any. She can read lips quite well, though. Just speak clearly for her.

Dory: (very loudly) Hi, Honey. I'm Dory. You can call me Grandma Dory.

Annie: (laughing) Dory, speaking clearly, not loudly. I'm afraid speaking loudly won't help. (signing) Emma, this is my sister, Millie.

Millie: Hello, Emma. Call me Aunt Millie. (they embrace) How'd I do?

Annie: Fine.

Millie: Emma, you also have an Uncle Kurt, and next summer you're going to have a little cousin!

Annie: What? Millie, that's marvelous!

Millie: Annie, quick, introduce her to Ethan.

Annie: Emma, this is my brother, your Uncle Ethan.

Ethan: Hey, squirt, you're cute. Don't you think I am?

Emma: (makes the sign for no)

Annie: That means no, Ethan.

Claudia: At least she's honest.

Annie: Yes, and she's very smart. You should see some of the pictures she draws. She's quite a little artist.

Claudia: (signs) Emma, Honey, am I beautiful?

Emmett: (nods her head)

Dory: You know how to speak to her!

Claudia: Yes, and I've brainwashed her. If you'll all act naturally this would be a lot easier.

Emmett: Well, Claudia, since you seem to know more about her than the rest of us, is there anything else we need to know?

Millie: Daddy!

Annie: I'm sorry. (walks with Emma over to Emmett) Emma, this is my father, your grandfather. Hello, Daddy.

Emmett: Hello, Ann.

(Emma pulls at her mother's arm.)

Annie: Yes?

Emma: (signs that she wants to know what to call him)

Annie: Oh, yes. She wants to know what to call you.

(The lights fade to dim and come up on a separately lit area. Enter young Mr. Westbrook.)

Young Emmett: Annie? Annie! Where are you? It's time for bed. Oh, I understand. (clears throat) Princess Ann. Princess Ann, the rest of your castle has gone to sleep. Is her excellency ready to retire?

Young Annie: Yes, Big Daddy.

Young Emmett: Tell me, Little Princess Ann, why do you call me Big Daddy?

Young Annie: Because you're my Daddy and because you're so big!

Young Emmett: Well, that makes sense to me. Good night, Princess Ann.

Young Annie: Good night, Big Daddy.

(The lights fade on them and come back up on the mainstage.)

Millie: Well, I think I should have something to say about what name we choose for you as a grandfather.

Ethan: Hey, I know! Dad, what was that name that Annie used to call you when she was little?

Emmett: I, uh, I don't think my memory is that good.

Annie: I remember, Daddy. I was your little Princess, and I called you Big Daddy.

Emmett: Yes.

Ethan: Big Daddy. That's right. Hey, that's a great name. How do I say it to her?

Annie: Like it sounds.

Ethan: Hey, Emma. (signs and talks simultaneously) Big Daddy! Can you do that? (Emma turns to Emmett and mimics the sign. They all laugh.)

Millie: Annie, she's so smart!

Claudia: Of course! She has inherited my memorization skills.

Dory: Claudia, you haven't changed a bit—you hate being upstaged by anyone! This food is gettin' cold. Let's eat. We've already thanked the Lord.

Millie: So, Claudia, have you won an Academy Award yet?

Claudia: No, Millicent Dear. Oscars are for movies and film in general, neither of which I choose to be involved with. Movie stars have no real talent.

Dory: Well, they must be doing something right—they're making more money than we do.

Claudia: True, but think of all they're missing. They have no audience, no interaction, no applause, no . . .

Dory: Egos?

(everyone laughs)

Claudia: Make fun if you will. But I work very hard to refine my craft. If I make a mistake on stage my audience sees. Therefore, I make none. If a film "star" makes an error, they simply stop the tape and take it again. There is no comparing film and stage talent.

Emmett: So, Claudia, tell us. Are you on or off-Broadway this month?

Claudia: Right now I am on!

Millie: For how long?

Claudia: Well, that depends on our success, Dear. So far we have been very successful. In fact, hold onto your hats—rumor has it that I will be nominated for a Tony this spring!

Dory: Now, is Tony any kin to Oscar?

Claudia: This is futile. Oscars are for film . . .

Dory: Oh, simmer down, I'm just pullin' your chain. I'm sure you're a fine actor.

Claudia: Thank you, Dory, Dear. And it's *actress*. Emmett, you've hardly said two words since I arrived. What's the matter, has the cat got your tongue?

Millie: Claudia, please!

Claudia: Millicent I'm too busy to fly in from New York just for small talk. Well, Emmett?

Emmett: Nothing is wrong with me, Claudia. I just don't have much to say to anyone, that's all.

(Annie, who has been cutting Emma's meat, knocks over a water glass.)

Annie: Oh, I'm sorry! I'm such a klutz lately. I'm sorry.

Claudia: How can you not have much to say to anyone? Two of your children haven't been here in nearly a year and Annie's been away for five!

Dory: It's all right, Sweetheart. Did the baby get wet?

Annie: No.

Claudia: Emmett!

Emmett: (stands) Claudia, what do you want me to say? My son comes home and after nine months still has no plans for his future. Millie tells me I'm going to be a grandfather again when I didn't feel like one to begin with. And Annie shows up, just shows up after five years with a grand-daughter I can't even speak to! It is obvious to me that I was coerced this morning into inviting you all here, so just what is it that you would like for me to say, hmmm?

(There is a long pause—then Emma tugs at her mother and signs something. Claudia begins to laugh.)

Annie: No, Emma, not now.

Ethan: What'd she say?

Annie: Drop it, Ethan.

Ethan: What? It's something funny. What does she think Dad should say?

(Everyone is laughing except Annie.)

Claudia: (has tried to maintain herself) Whew! Out of the mouths of babes! Ha! It seems to be the opinion of this child, Emmett, that you . . . say you are sorry and then go to your room. (Everyone laughs, even Annie. When they realize Emmett is not amused, they stop.)

Emmett: I see. (clears throat) Well, Emma, since this is your first visit to my house, I apologize. I behaved badly. I think I'll retire now.

Annie: Oh no, Daddy. Don't. She was just repeating what I've said to her before. She didn't mean it.

Emmett: No, I uh, I have to pack. I'm flying into Chicago Sunday. I promised Lyndon.

Dory: (suspicious) You didn't mention any trip to me. It's Christmas!

Emmett: Dorothy, Monday is Christmas, and I'll be back before then. I'm flying in and back out on Sunday. This new contract needs my signature. It's fine with me if you stay the weekend. (pause) Good night. (exits)

Scene Six

Claudia: Hmph! Wasn't that big of him!

Annie: It's OK, Claudia. He did ask us to stay, at least.

Ethan and Millie: Yes.

Claudia: Is that what you think? Is that what you think he said? 'Cause he didn't! He said, "It's fine with me if you stay the weekend." That's all! Who needs permission to stay in their own house? (long pause) Nobody! That's who! Hmph! And to think of all the years I've been missing out on the merriment of having a family of my own!

Annie: Claudia, Daddy mentioned a new contract. Now, I'm sure he's just under tremendous pressure.

Claudia: Is that really what you all think?

Millie: Maybe not, but he's our father, and we need to honor his wishes.

Ethan: You'd understand if you knew him better, Claudia.

Claudia: May I remind you that I have known him longer than any of you—since we were kids? If it weren't for me he'd never have met your mother and *none* of you would *even* be sitting here!

Dory: OK, Claudia. We are eternally grateful to you. Let's just eat. (Everyone resumes eating and Claudia just stares at them.)

Claudia: I don't believe this. I don't. Your mother has created little monsters out of all of you!

All: What?!

Claudia: Grace Westbrook was the most forgiving, understanding person I've ever known and unfortunately, you're all just like her!

Millie: Claudia, let's finish dinner, and then we'll discuss it. OK?

Claudia: No, Millie, it is not OK. Because, we will finish dinner, we'll all go to bed, and the subject will never come up until next Christmas, or the next Easter, or even worse, at one of your funerals! Your father needs a loving confrontation, not your tolerance. You seem to think you'll keep him happy by keeping quiet. Well (pause), does he look happy to you? He looks like "The Grinch Who Stole Christmas" to me!

Millie: You're right, Claudia. Mother did much more than just tolerate something—she tried to correct it. Do you really think we should confront Daddy?

Claudia: I said *lovingly* confront him—there's a difference. However, you might consider tying him up first.

Ethan: We could do it tomorrow before he leaves town on Sunday. We'll just sit down and have a family talk. What do you think, Annie?

Annie: I don't think I want to.

Ethan: Oh, come on, it'll be as easy as when we used to gang up on Dad to get our way when Dory first came.

Dory: Ethan!

Ethan: Sorry.

Millie: Count me in. I think a family talk is long overdue. Come on, Annie, this isn't like you. What's wrong?

Annie: It's just that I had made plans with Claudia to take Emma shopping tomorrow for Christmas gifts. Then we'll have to come home and open presents right after that, is all.

Millie: (confused) Emma, tomorrow is Saturday. You know Daddy doesn't allow us to open gifts until Christmas Eve.

Annie: Since when?

Ethan: Since the year we tried it and complained we didn't have anything to open when Christmas Eve came. Annie, do you feel all right?

Annie: Of course I do, don't be silly! I'm all right! I just got my days mixed up. Plus, I've been trying to slow down a little too. Sometimes when I plan too much in one day I tend to forget things. Everybody does that.

Millie: Annie, we're trying to plan a little discussion, not a family vacation. Can't you help us talk to Dad after you shop?

Annie: Of course, I can. I'll write it down, and I'll be there.

Ethan: (winks) Thanks for squeezing us in, Sis.

Dory: Hey, everyone, the family talk is set for tomorrow. Now leave Annie alone. She's tired and under a lot of pressure. It's tough trying to be both Mama and Daddy at the same time.

Claudia: And how would you know about that?

Dory: I know firsthand from watchin' their father try it—you remember.

Claudia: Yes, I do.

Millie: Oh, how I do wish Mother were here now to see Emma and our baby. I think she would have been as good of a Grandma as she was a mother.

Ethan: Annie, you're a good mom. I'm so happy to finally meet Emma.

Annie: I'm sorry, very sorry to all of you. I've missed you terribly even though I've stayed away. I've missed Daddy most of all. At first I was so angry that he wouldn't accept Jeff that it was easy for me to stay away. Then when Emma came along a year later, everything changed. Things looked different to me. I wanted her to have everything, especially a grandfather.

Millie: Why didn't you just tell Daddy that?

Annie: I tried. But Daddy and I are too much alike. We both talk really well and listen very poorly. There's something you need to remember too. If now is the time for Daddy and me to restore our relationship, it won't be because Daddy suddenly realized how wrong he might have been. And it won't be because I've had a child and have some new insight as to how wrong I might have been. It will be because we love and miss each other very much. I want that to be the reason when we forgive each other.

Dory: Well, I think that's the best reason!

Annie: I appreciated all of your letters. They have really brought me out of some heavy depressions.

Ethan: I have never known you to be depressed, Annie.

Annie: Well, I have been a lot. It was Jeff's major complaint, but I am approaching it prayerfully. I need to get past that. Coming here will help, I just know it. I feel more relaxed right now than I have in years.

Millie: Well, it's no wonder. New York has got to be the most unrelaxing place to live.

Annie: No, not really. Claudia thinks we should be roommates.

Dory: Now *that* would be unrelaxing!

Annie: No, she's hardly ever home.

Dory: That's what I hear. I understand you have many friends. *Men* friends, I mean.

Claudia: (crosses to rocking chair) Dory, just because I'm middle aged and have never married does not mean I behave improperly.

Dory: Middle aged?! Ha! Do you plan on living to be 110?

Claudia: Yes, I do! All right, so I'll never be a mother. How do you know I'd make a good one, or that I even wanted to be one? Some people just know themselves well enough to be honest. (pause) And honestly, I guess I did want to be a mother deep down inside. I just got too busy being everything else. Funny, your mother never *wanted* to be anything else.

(Abruptly, a young Claudia Carney appears on the other stage dressed in ballet-wear. She is searching for young Grace.)

Young Claudia: Grace! Grace! Where are you? We're supposed to be rehearsing.

Young Grace: I'm coming, Claudia. I'm coming as fast as I can. (she enters)

Young Claudia: Oh no, you're not. You're trying to quit on me!

Young Grace: Claudia, we've been practicing too long. I'm tired.

Claudia: Practice makes perfect, you know!

Young Grace: Well, then, you should be perfect by now. I'll never be. I'm too clumsy.

Young Claudia: No, you're not! Grace, it's just that thing you have—that disease. I keep trying to tell you that if you'll just tighten your shoes and work really hard you'll make it go away. Please try.

Young Grace: Claudia, it's not ever going to go away. It's only going to get worse.

Young Claudia: Stop that talk, Grace Ann Murray. Don't you want to grow up and be famous like moi?

Grace: No, not really.

Young Claudia: Well, what do you want to be?

Grace: I want to be a mother.

Young Claudia: (in disgust) Oooh! A mother?! I don't know any really beautiful mothers. That's not a very glamorous job.

Young Grace: Sure it is. Your children look to you for everything, and they think you're the most beautiful person in the world.

Young Claudia: Beautiful, huh? Hey, maybe you've got something there. Kids would be a captive audience. Hey, are you rested up now?

Young Grace: (surprised) I think I am!

Young Claudia: Good. Let's go into my bedroom and rehearse to music. And this time, no falling down!

Young Grace: OK, Claudia. I'll try.

(They run off and the lights come back upon mainstage.)

Dory: Well, I can't sit here all night. I guess I'd better take these dishes we've cleared and wash them. Claudia, could you help out? (There is no response.) Claudia!

Claudia: Hmm? Oh, I'm sorry. I was just remembering something.

Ethan: Come on, Dory, you wash and I'll dry.

Millie: I'll help too but then I'm going to bed. I'm exhausted . . .

Annie: Millie, you need your rest. Go to bed. I'll help, Dory. Could you put Emma to bed for me?

Claudia: No, uh, Annie, could I put Emma to bed tonight?

Annie: Sure, she'd like that. Did you draw this, Emma? It's beautiful. May I have it? Thank you. Goodnight, Sweety.

(Everyone exits except Claudia and Emma.)

Claudia: Emma, come here. I want you to meet someone. (shows picture) This is your grandmother. Her name was Grace.

Emma: (makes the sign for beautiful)

Claudia: Yes, she was beautiful, and she'd be happy that you thought so. She was the most godly woman, the most godly *person* I ever knew.

That's what made her beautiful. *That's* what *kept* her beautiful. (reaching for Emma) Come here, Baby. (begins to rock) I'd sing to you, but it wouldn't do any good, would it? I could also recite Shakespeare, but that wouldn't impress you either. (sighs) Aren't we a funny pair? All I know how to do is talk, and all you know how to do is love. You can't hear a word I say, but you understand me better than anyone. I am sure of that. (Emma has gone to sleep, but she continues to rock and recites.)

> Birds of a feather flock together,
> And so will pigs and swine;
> Ducks and geese will have their choice
> And so, I will have mine.

(She kisses Emma, and the lights go down on the sound of a chair rocking.)

END OF ACT ONE

ACT TWO

Scene One

(Enter Mr. Westbrook dressed in a suit. He is carrying a briefcase. He sets it down at the table, pours a cup of coffee, and begins searching for some papers.)

Emmett: OK, Dorothy, where is my contract? (He keeps searching and Dorothy enters a moment later, obviously angry at him.)

Dory: Oh, there you are.

Emmett: (sweetly, with a scheme) Good morning, Dorothy. Say, you haven't happened to see my contract that was lying here yesterday, have you?

Dory: Maybe I have, and maybe I haven't.

Emmett: I see. Is there some reason that you don't want to tell me?

Dory: Maybe there is, and maybe there isn't.

Emmett: Are you planning on destroying the contract?

Dory: (slyly) Maybe I am, and maybe I'm not.

Emmett: Dorothy, are you ever going to stop talking in these rhymes?

Dory: (glaring) No.

Emmett: OK, I give up. Just roll up your sleeves and hit me with your best shot.

(Dory advances to him and rolls up her sleeves.)

Emmett: Are you really going to hit me?

Dory: I should! Oh boy, I'd love to! But, no. You see, I have washed my hands clean of you.

Emmett: In what sense?

Dory: (in his face) I am saying that for once and for all, Emmett Lee Westbrook, I have turned *you* over to the Lord!

Emmett: Dorothy, I have obviously upset you. Now please tell me what I have done, and I will discuss it with you calmly. Just hurry please before I have a flight to catch.

Dory: That is what's the matter with me. *That* is what's wrong with your children *and* now your grandchildren. Get over here—you've got lint all over you.

Emmett: What?

(Dory goes to a drawer and gets some masking tape. As she speaks she stretches and wraps the tape around her hand and then crosses to him. She begins removing the lint by slapping his back with her hand gently at first. Then as she becomes angrier she gets rougher with him.)

Dory: After Mrs. Grace died all the children ever needed was *you*. They didn't need a big fancy house, fancy clothes, fancy toys, or even a fancy education. They wouldn't have *even* needed me. But you buried yourself in your writing and left those younguns' for me to raise. All by myself. And I stayed all these years 'cause I enjoyed feelin' needed like that. But I don't enjoy it no more. (hard slap)

Emmett: (interrupting) Ow! Dorothy!

Dory: Sit down! (She pushes him down in a chair and starts working on his pant legs. She is lifting his legs as she speaks, slapping him harder and harder, even hitting his reflexes.) Your children mustered up all the courage they had and asked you to join them in a simple family discussion yesterday. And you had the nerve to tell them you were too busy!

Emmett: I was!

Dory: You could've made the time. And after you turned them down what'd they say? "OK, Daddy, we understand how busy you are." I have no clue, I say, no clue as to why your children keep forgiving you. Probably 'cause Mrs. Grace took 'em to church and taught 'em so. You "oughta" be a grateful man. I say, grateful.

Emmett: Dorothy, I am grateful. However, we are going to have to postpone this chat. My plane leaves in a few minutes.

(Dorothy pauses and looks at him with disgust, then asks slyly . . .)

Dory: What time is it, Sir?

Emmett: Well, to be exact it is . . . (He reaches into his pocket for his pocket watch. While his hands are busy she quickly opens a wide strip of tape and begins winding it around him rapidly, tying him to the chair.) Dorothy! What in the world are you doing? I'll miss my flight! (She ignores him.) Dorothy, stop it. Dorothy. Dorothy! Uh, Dorothy, I think Emma is calling you. *Why are you doing this?*

Dory: Emma is why I'm doin' this.

(He relaxes and they pause.)

Emmett: I thought you turned me over to the Lord.

Dory: I did. But if I were Him I wouldn't want to have anything to do with you!

Emmett: Lucky for me you're not Him.

Dory: Sir, just for a moment I want you to look upon me not just as an employee, but as a friend.

Emmett: (looks at the tape on himself) It will be difficult, but I will try.

Dory: Your children keep coming back around even when you don't seem to care. It's probably been years since you've even looked one of 'em in the eye and said you loved 'em. Now Emma's here. I saw how you looked at that baby when she stepped in here the other night. I did. And I knew just what you were thinkin'! You were thinkin' about how much she looked like Miss Annie when she was little. Don't deny it. She's the spittin' image of Annie, and you noticed it! But how is Emma gonna know you love her, Sir, if you don't look her in the eye and say it? Her eyes are all she has!

Emmett: Thank you for your honesty, Dorothy. I see your point. (pauses and chooses his words carefully, not wanting to upset her again) Are we through now?

Dory: Yes. I am now turning you back over to the Lord.

Emmett: Could you untie me now, please?

Dory: Are you going to Chicago?

Emmett: Maybe I will, and maybe I won't. (Dory briefly stops untying him.) I'm joking! Since it's Christmas Eve, I won't go. Are you happy?

Dory: Almost.

Emmett: What would make you totally happy?

Dory: A nice family Christmas around a nice little tree.

Emmett: I'll see what I can do.

Dory: Good. Well, seein' as how you're all cleaned up—no lint and everything—I want us all to go to church this morning.

Emmett: Now that I've missed my flight I'm going to have to go to into the office and call Lyndon. Dory, I know that it's Christmas, but . . .

Dory: No. I don't want you to go because it's Christmas. I just want you to go because it's Sunday.

Emmett: I'll go to the office first and then try to meet you all at church, OK?

Dory: OK, here are yesterday's newspapers.

Emmett: No thank you, but may I please have my contract now?

(She goes to the freezer, takes it out, and hands it to him.)

Emmett: Let's hope it thaws in time for church. Good-bye. (Claudia enters.)

Dory: Good-bye sir. I enjoyed our talk.

Claudia: Good morning, Dory. Is that Emmett leaving?

Dory: Yes, but he's gonna meet us at church, Claudia!

Claudia: How can you be sure?

Dory: Well, he said he'd try. He'd better be there, or I'm gonna tie him up again.

Claudia: What? You tied Emmett up?

Dory: Yep. (shows her the wad of tape) I gave him a piece of my mind too.

Claudia: Well, Dorothy Oakes, I knew there was something I liked about you! What'd you say to him?

Dory: I told him . . . you want some coffee? (pours) I told him he'd better fix his wagon before those kids of his gave up on him. I told him to do it especially for Emma.

Claudia: I never knew you had it in you. I'm glad you do.

Dory: We're not so different, you and me. (pauses) Neither of us ever married.

Claudia: No.

Dory: Or had children . . .

Claudia: No.

Dory: We're both far too outspoken.

Claudia: True, true. (They both sigh deeply.) But, you know, Dory, there is one more thing.

Dory: What's that?

Claudia: We're both strikingly beautiful.

Dory: Really? (She seems pleased.) Thank you, Claudia. That's the nicest thing you ever said to me. (stands) I'll just go up now and touch up my makeup before church. Thanks again! (mumbles) Strikingly beautiful . . . ha! . . . who'd have guessed it?

Scene Two

(Enter Annie somewhat dressed for church with her hair very messy.)

Annie: Morning, Claudia. Any clues as to why Dory is in such a good mood?

Claudia: Yes, we had a chat. Hey, aren't you going to church with us? Your dad's going to try and be there.

Annie: Of course, I'm going. Why?

Claudia: Well, Honey, pardon me for saying so, but I felt the urge to hum the death march when you walked in.

Annie: Feel free. It would match my mood.

Claudia: Honey, you can't be depressed today. It's Christmas Eve! The whole family is going to church, and then there's dinner and presents!

Annie: I know.

Claudia: Is it because your dad wouldn't talk through things yesterday?

Annie: I don't know.

Claudia: Well, you've got to know what's bothering you. If you don't know, who does?

Annie: Look, Claudia. I know I shouldn't be down, but for some strange reason I am, OK?

Claudia: OK, honey, just make up your mind—depression or anger.

Annie: I'm sorry, Claudia. (pauses) Is that decaf?

Claudia: Yes. Would you like a donut too?

Annie: (simply nods her head)

Claudia: (has poured) You take two scoops, right?

Annie: Yes. (has taken a bite of the donut but is having trouble swallowing)

Claudia: What's wrong?

Annie: My throat. I can hardly swallow.

Claudia: (feeling her head) Is it sore?

Annie: No, not really. I'll just drink this.

Claudia: Are you sure you're not sick? We can stay home, you know.

Annie: No, I feel like going. Really.

Claudia: OK, but we've got to do something with your appearance and quick. Do you have a brush and some pins?

Annie: I think so.

Claudia: I'll just brush it all up and twist it around here. It'll be up now, so you'll need some earrings.

Annie: No, that's OK.

Claudia: (confused) All right. Give me a pin. (She notices Annie is trembling.) Annie, you're trembling!

Annie: I am not.

Claudia: Yes, you are. I saw your hand tremble just now.

Annie: I'm just hungry. Hurry up or we're going to be late.

Claudia: Give me another pin.

Annie: That's all I have.

Claudia: Well, it's not going to stay. We'll have to stop by Barry's 24-hour Drug Store and get some pretty combs. Got any lipstick? (Annie hands it over.) Open. Girl, you look peaked! When we get back from church you're going straight up to bed. Understand?

Annie: Why, yes, Mammy. And would you like for me to pinch my cheeks and make them rosy too?

Claudia: Fine. Make fun of me for trying to take care of you.

Annie: What are you doing?

Claudia: I'm leaving Millie a note to tell her that we went on ahead. I'm also asking Dory to dress Emma.

Annie: I'll be in the car. (She exits.)
(enter Ethan)

Ethan: Good morning and Merry Christmas Eve!

Claudia: Ethan, do be a dear and give this to Millie. Also, would you drive everyone else to church?

Ethan: Sure, but wait. Where are you going?

Claudia: I'm taking Annie shopping at the drug store.

Ethan: On Sunday?

Claudia: Yes. She was so depressed this morning that she barely dressed herself. I thought a new hairdo might perk her up, though. We'll meet you there, Babe. Thanks. (exits, then reappears) Oh, Ethan, Merry Christmas to you too.

Scene Three

(Ethan crosses to the coffee maker and discovers it is empty. Instead, he pours some orange juice and eats a donut. He reaches over to the mail stack, glances at a paper, and then sees the HD envelope. He cleans his hands and opens it, spilling several brochures, letters, and booklets. Picks up newsletter and reads article.) "BEFORE YOU SIGN" please think about asking your attorney to include an additional paragraph in your will—a paragraph making a bequest to the Huntington's Disease Society of America. (turns page) "LIVING WITH HD" (turns page) "GENETIC BREAKTHROUGHS IN HD" (turns page) "SYMPTOMS OF HD" (turns page) "HAVING YOUR FAMILY TESTED FOR THE HD GENE" (He looks confused and turns back to the article on symptoms of HD. Silently, he reads fast and furiously as he scans through the literature and realizes that Annie has displayed these symptoms. Reads aloud now.) The first symptoms of Huntington's Disease may be clumsiness, dropping objects, or restlessness. Personality changes may be noted such as mood swings or *depression.* This often leads to a carelessness about personal grooming. Most patients lose their capacity to plan, organize, and sequence daily affairs as before, and even find it difficult to maintain routine appointments. As the disease progresses, walking becomes difficult because muscle spasms cause jerking and twitching. In an early onset, however, the movements may be slower, and may resemble trembling. The disease gradually destroys the patient's intellect and memory and results in death some ten to fifteen years later. HD is a severe hereditary disorder of the nervous system. Symptoms in most cases begin between the ages of 30 and 50, but have been reported as early as age two and as late as age 70. (reads rapidly) Each child of a patient with HD has a 50 percent chance of inheriting the gene. If you carry the gene, you will develop the disease if you live long enough, AND, YOU CAN PASS IT ON. (He sits back and stares ahead, then covers his eyes with his hands. The lights fade on mainstage, and at the same time on the alternate stage, a young Ethan Westbrook is heard screaming. A young Emmett Westbrook enters carrying the screaming boy. Young Millicent also enters with her arm around a young Annie. They are dressed as if they are returning from a funeral.)

Young Ethan: Mommy! Mommy! I want my Mommy! Let me see her!

Young Emmett: Ethan! Stop it. Stop it now. (He holds the boy close to him and finally the boy stops screaming and relaxes in his arms. He cries softly.) Ethan, everything is going to get better. You'll see. Ssh. We have each other still.

Millie: Daddy, are you going to get sick and leave us too?

Young Emmett: No, Honey. HD doesn't work that way. It's not contagious.

Young Millie: Then we won't get it either?

Young Emmett: (chooses his words very carefully) Well, Millicent . . . there is a 50 percent chance you could, because HD is hereditary.

Annie: What is hereditary?

Ethan: Hereditary is when you look like someone.

Young Emmett: Yes, Ethan, and sometimes people in the same family look alike on the inside too. Mommy was sick on the inside ever since she was a little girl. She was younger than any of you when she got HD. We don't know that much about the disease yet, but I figure since you're all so healthy, maybe you've outsmarted it, huh? Let's not think about that right now.

Young Millie: Daddy, where is Mommy now?

Young Emmett: (pauses) She's walking in heaven, Millicent. She's walking easily . . . gracefully too. And her insides are all better, Ethan.

Young Ethan: Then I'm glad that she's there.

(The father holds his arms out and the children embrace him—the lights fade and come back upon mainstage where Ethan is still sitting. He uncovers his face and sighs, then continues looking through the rest of the literature. Millie enters.)

Millie: Good morning, Ethan. Have you looked outside? It's snowing!

Ethan: Millie, did Annie ever get tested for HD?

Millie: Well, no. Unlike us, she didn't want to know if she was carrying the gene. Why?

Ethan: Everything makes sense now.

Millie: Ethan, what are you talking about?

Ethan: What year were you and I tested?

Millie: Well, it was the year after the genetic marker was discovered, so it would've been 1984. Why?

Ethan: Emma. Annie was pregnant with Emma in 1984 and said she didn't want to be tested. But she suspected it then, and that's why she stayed away so willingly. (pause) She's got it, Millie, and she's known about it since Emma was born.

Millie: Why doesn't she want us to find out?

Ethan: She doesn't want to find out herself, don't you see? Once she's told for sure she has the gene, that means Emma may carry it also.

Millie: Ethan, you're scaring me.

Ethan: Millie, don't be frightened. You don't carry the gene. Neither do I. We can't pass it on to our kids.

Millie: But if Annie has it she can?

Ethan: Early symptoms listed here are slurred speech, depression, clumsiness, restlessness, forgetfulness, nervousness . . .

Millie: But Ethan, she's had good reason to be nervous with the tension between her and Daddy—nerves would cause any of those symptoms. And besides, I remember what Mom went through better than you do. Annie doesn't have any of those physical symptoms.

Ethan: But that's the nature of the disease. It attacks mental abilities first. Besides, you remember Mom in the final stage of her disease. Annie may be in the first stage—the symptoms progress, Millie. Look, let's back up a minute. Mom had juvenile HD—she got it as a kid. It says here that juvenile HD may display different symptoms from regular Huntington's.

Millie: I thought all this was behind us. Now it's starting all over again.

Ethan: Millicent, don't do this. You've got to help me talk to Dad and get some information. We need to get a doctor over here that knows about HD, one that can recognize it.

Millie: What about Dr. Grayson? He's the one who correctly diagnosed Mom. He'd know.

Ethan: Is he still in Brookport?

Millicent: I think so. And he'd be happy to come under the circumstances. Do you want me to call him now?

Ethan: No. Annie's not even here; neither is Dad. And we can't just have a doctor waiting here for her when she gets back. Look, let's just calmly get Dory and Emma in the car and meet the others at church.

Millie: I'll ride home alone with Annie and talk to her then. You try to talk to Dad, OK? (He nods.) I remember when we were kids and Mom got so sick right before she died; I prayed everyday, "God, please make her better, and please let them find a cure." (turns to him) Ethan, is it wrong to pray for a healing, when the healing may not be in God's will?

Ethan: Millicent, it's never wrong to pray, and it's never too late for a healing. (They join hands, bow their heads, and the lights fade.)

Scene Four

(Enter Dory carrying a tray of food. She places it on the table and snacks from it nervously. She sits and waits, then stands and rearranges the food on the table several times. Claudia enters and Dory stands.)

Dory: Any word yet?

Claudia: Not a peep. This sure is a nice spread.

Dory: Well, you look hungry so come on over and eat a bit. I figured the family dinner would be canceled so I just whipped up some finger foods. No sense in anybody starving!

Claudia: Dory, nobody's going to starve as long as you're around.

Dory: I suppose. You know, I keep picturing Annie gettin' real sick like her mother did. It makes me real sad. And then there's Emma. What's going to become of her? Do you think her father will take her in?

Claudia: No, and I wouldn't want him to either. If he walked out once, he just might do it again.

Dory: Emma will need special care. Special schooling.

Claudia: We're getting ahead of ourselves, Dory. We don't even know if it's HD yet.

(Enter Ethan.)

Ethan: Oh, food! Dory, how did you know I was hungry?

Claudia: She doesn't have to be a genius to know that you're always hungry. It's probably your nerves that are making you hungry. Funny, stress makes me lose my appetite.

Dory: Hmph! I wish it made me lose mine. When are they comin' down? I can't eat much more!

Claudia: They've been up there two hours.

Ethan: Dr. Grayson said the preliminary evaluation would take a while. Pass me some of that dip, please.

(Enter Dr. Grayson and Millie. The rest stand.)

Claudia: Martin, what do you think?

Dr. Grayson: Everyone, be seated, I need to talk with you. Where is Emmett?

Claudia: He was supposed to meet us at church, but he never did. He should be here soon.

Dr. Grayson: I'd rather not discuss this in his absence, but I know you have all been waiting. First, let me say that a bedside evaluation will not be sufficient to make a correct diagnosis of HD. I'm going to need to run an MRI scan and a computed tomography. We'll also need to get bloodwork.

Millicent: Doctor, we have a family history of this disease. So, it's something we've always considered. Just tell us now what your first impression is of Annie's condition.

Dr. Grayson: Your mother was the first HD patient I treated. In a town the size of Brookport you don't see many cases of it, partially because people deny this disease. It's not pretty. But your mother had been told since childhood that she had another neurological disorder—benign familial chorea. It wasn't until the disease began to progress rapidly that she started coming to me. By the time I correctly diagnosed it as HD, it was too late. She had already run the risk of passing the gene on to one of you. I'll be honest, though. Even if your mother had known she had Huntington's, I believe she still would have had all three of you. Unfortunately, it is my opinion that the HD gene *was* passsed on to Annie.

Ethan: Where do we go from here? What's next?

Dr. Grayson: Well, there are five stages of the disease and from what I've seen today, I believe she is in stage two. Extensive testing should begin soon, but it can wait until after the holidays. After that, I'm going to suggest some counseling—I know you can go to your pastor. I also feel that you should be around other HD families. Unfortunately, the nearest support group is two hours away in St. Louis.

Millie: That's where we live!

Dr. Grayson: Ethan, Millie tells me that you both tested negative for the defective gene. HD does not skip generations. If you don't get it you can't pass it on.

Ethan: Yes, sir.

Dr. Grayson: There's so much more you need to know, and it cannot be crammed into one afternoon. I suggest you contact the HD Society of America.

Claudia: Yes, we will. But in a moment Annie is going to walk through that door, and we need to know what to do. We need to know what to say.

Dr. Grayson: You need to say Merry Christmas, Annie, or whatever you would say to her on any given Sunday afternoon. What I mean is: be yourselves. Annie will feel better if she's happy. When she experiences great stress her symptoms will appear more severe.

Millie: If she has HD, are there any medications she can take?

Dr. Grayson: Twenty years ago when someone was diagnosed with HD, we put them on Haldol. That's what your mother took. But it only suppresses certain symptoms. We may try a brief trial, but if I see that the medicinal side-effects are worse than her original symptoms, then it's hard to argue that it's worth taking the medicine at all.

Dr. Grayson: There is one thing that seems to help.

All: What?

Dr. Grayson: Nutritional studies have shown that patients who don't get too thin seem to do better. Most patients need between 4,000 and 6,000 calories daily.

Dory: I can help there! I know all her favorite foods. I'll get that girl plump, you'll see!

Claudia: Well, you've made Dory happy.

Doctor: I'm going to go now, but I'll be in touch. Remember nobody dies *of* Huntington's Disease—they die *with* it. This will be gradual, so help Annie to get on with what's left of her life. Try and have a Merry Christmas.

Claudia: You, too. Thank you for coming. Good-bye.

Ethan: Well, how do we act normal?

Dory: Well, I've got some wrapping to finish up so I think I'll go do that. You promise me that you'll all eat?

All: Yes, Dory.

Dory: I'll be upstairs if you need more food.

Millicent: Ethan, I have a wonderful idea.

Ethan: What?

Millie: Emma will be up from her nap soon. Why don't we go up in the attic and get the Christmas decorations down?

Claudia: Oh, she'd love that!

Millie: Yes, and Dory said Daddy was going to try and find a tree for us.

(enter Emmett)

Scene Five

Claudia: So much for the tree! Where have you been?

Emmett: I got tied up. Again.

Claudia: Yes, and it's going to be for a third time if you don't straighten up. Only this time you're all mine.

Ethan: Claudia, this won't help matters.

Claudia: Funny, sure helps me feel better! I'm going to get Emma up from her nap.

Ethan: Dad, we need to talk.

Emmett: You sound as if something is wrong.

Millie: It is, Daddy. It's about Annie.

Ethan: Whatever differences Annie and I may have are none of your concern.

Millie: Daddy, it's not that. I wish it were that simple.

Ethan: Dad, we think Annie has . . . Huntington's.

(Emmett says nothing, but takes a seat front and center.)

Millie: We've all noticed the symptoms but didn't really recognize them. Ethan found this literature this morning and, well, the more he read, the more it made sense.

Ethan: We called Mart Grayson, and he came and stayed for a couple of hours. He examined Annie, and he does think it's HD. (Ethan and Millie look at each other, wondering why Emmett doesn't respond.) Of course, they'll need more tests.

Millie: Daddy, he thinks Annie is already at stage two.

(enter Annie)

Ethan: Hey, squirt, you OK?

Annie: (nods yes)

Millie: Ethan, why don't we go get those Christmas decorations? We'll be in the attic. (They leave slowly.)

Annie: We missed you at church this morning, Daddy. Emma loved her Sunday School class, but then, she fits in well wherever she goes. She drew you a picture—you've made quite an impression on her, you know. She loves her big Daddy. (pause) Daddy, I need to tell you something and it's very important. But before we get into that we need to work things out between us. I don't even know where to start. I'm sure it all began over Jeff, and perhaps you were right about him. But, I need your forgiveness, Daddy. (pause) And if I've hurt you in any other way . . . or not lived up to what you expected of me . . . I am sorry, Daddy. I'm sorry, Daddy! I miss you, Daddy. (She turns to leave and spills a dish, then begins to yell with slurred speech.) I don't kn-kn-know what you w-w-want from me, but I know what I want f-f-from you. (shouts & cries) I need my f-father. And I will not allow you to push me away from you! (She drops to the floor over the dish she has spilled. Emmett, totally broken in spirit and on the verge of tears, rushes to her side, grabbing her by the shoulders and lifts her up. They stare at each other for a moment, then embrace quickly.)

Emmett: (slowly) Oh, Annie . . . I am so sorry. I don't want to push you away. I want us to be close, like we used to be. (He looks at her.) And you don't need my forgiveness. I need yours. I ask you—no, I beg you—for it. I am going to change. I need your help, and I need your prayers, but you have my word. We're going to make the most of what's left.

Annie: You know.

Emmett: Ethan and Millie told me. Annie, if I could I'd make it all go away. How I wish there was something they could take from me, and give to you. But they can't. And perhaps I've caused you more pain than HD ever will, so please Annie, take from me—a new heart. I love you, Princess.

Annie: I love you . . . Big Daddy.

(They hug and the lights fade on a quiet stage.)

Scene Six

(Enter Dory carrying a tray of monkey bread.)

Dory: Merry Christmas, Dory! Oh, this is the best Christmas I can remember. It is glorious having a child in the house—even Santa Clause has come! Oh it looks like Kurt sent Millie some Christmas roses. 1-2-3-4-5-6-7-8-9-10-11-12-13-14-15-16-17-18-19-20! (smells) My! How lovely! What? These are for me! (Quickly opens card) "I thank you for twenty years of friendship and loyalty, and, of course, the thousands of home-cooked meals. Which reminds me—how would you like to help me fulfill my new contract by writing me a #1 best-seller cookbook? With heartfelt thanks, Emmett." (She puts the card away and begins wiping her eyes on her apron.)

(enter Millie)

Millie: Merry Christmas, Dory—what's wrong?

Dory: Oh, Millie, I am 56 years old, and I've just received my first roses.

Millie: Really? Anybody I know?

Dory: Yes, he's upstairs asleep.

Millie: Dory!

Dory: Oh, silly girl. I mean your father. Your father has sent me Christmas roses.

Millie: Dory, I have only one father, and I don't think he's capable of such generosity. Are you sure you read the card right?

Dory: Yes, maybe the old Emmett Westbrook wouldn't do this, but the new and improved one would! I can't believe it! Of course, I should. I've been prayin' for that man for twenty years. Yes sir, pray without ceasin'; that's what I've been doin'. I can't believe it, but I do! I do, I do, I do, I do!

(enter Ethan with Christmas decorations)

Ethan: You do what, Dory?

Dory: I do believe this is the best Christmas ever!

Ethan: You're absolutely right! Now, three guesses as to what I found in the attic.

Millie: Hmm. Let's see. Is it that windup Santa doll?

Dory: No, Millie. Remember, Ethan wound him up too tight that one year, and he popped his head off.

Millie: Oh, that's right. Oh, I bet you found Dory's Elvis Presley *Blue Christmas* album.

Dory: Couldn't be. He stays down here with me year round. I just love that last song on Side A—"Mama Loved the Roses."

Millie: Did you find our old Christmas stockings?

Ethan: Yes, but that's not it. I found the Nativity scene! Remember, the one Dad used to help us set up every Christmas morning?

Millie: Oh, Ethan, I do remember! It's so dusty, though.

Dory: We'll clean it off and let Emma set it up later.

(enter Claudia and Emma)

Claudia: Well, good morning, everybody. Have you all noticed that we have a white Christmas?

Dory: Yes, and a Christmas angel too. Come here, Emma. What do you have here?

Claudia: She has been diligently working all morning. She has drawn you all special pictures for Christmas.

(Emma goes and hands each of them a picture, then runs back to Claudia.)

Millie: Emma, this is me! And this must be Kurt—you'll get to meet him later today!

Ethan: Look, she drew me too. And who's this beautiful woman beside me?

Dory: Dream on! That's Emma. These are amazing! How can she do this?

Claudia: Pretty incredible, huh?

Millie: Emma, I think there's something special for you right over here.

Ethan: Is Annie coming down?

Claudia: She's resting now, but I'm sure she will later. She and your father were up pretty late talking.

Millie: I am so happy that she and Daddy worked through everything. She certainly has a lot ahead of her now.

Claudia: It's odd, though, she didn't say a word about it this morning. She seemed happier and healthier than I've seen her in years.

Ethan: Where's Dad? Have any of you seen him?

Dory: No, and I've been up for quite a while baking this monkey bread— ya'll come eat up.

(enter Emmett covered with snow)

Emmett: Merry Christmas, everyone!

All: Daddy! Emmett! Where have you been?

Dory: You must have gotten up before I did this morning!

Emmett: Well, I never really went to bed. I decided just to stay up and go to the sunrise service at the church. (They are all silent.) Oh, wait here! (He exits and re-enters with a Christmas tree.)

All: Daddy, a tree!

Millie: Oh, Daddy. It's beautiful. Thank you.

Ethan: Let's decorate it.

Claudia: Emma, look at our tree. Come help us. (They all gather around and decorate.)

Dory: Sir, thank you for my roses. I was deeply touched.

Emmett: Dory, you're very welcome. Have you considered my offer?

Dory: Yes sir, and I'm flattered. Merry Christmas.

Emmett: Merry Christmas, Dory.

(From far away carolers begin to sing "Silent Night." Holding candles they approach the Westbrook house and stand outside the door. Everyone notices except Emma.)

Claudia: Listen!

Millie: We have some carolers!

Ethan: Hey, let's go join them.

(They bundle up quickly and go out to join the carolers who hand each of them a candle. As Ethan, Millie, Claudia, and Dory all become part of the carolers, they continue to sing softly. Emmett, on mainstage, turns to

Emma who is drawing with her new sketch set, and realizes she has not heard the carolers. He goes to her.)

Emmett: Princess, come here. I need your help. You see, I have a problem. I have to write two books this year. Now, I've taken care of one of them, but I need to come up with one more. Now, if I wrote a nifty little children's book, do you think you could find the time to illustrate it? (realizing she doesn't understand) Oh, let's see—(picks up crayons and sketch pad) Draw the pictures. Could you do that? See, (he writes) written by Emmett Lee Westbrook and illustrated by Emma Lee Scott. (She marks on the paper.) OK, OK, you'll get top billing—could you do that? (She nods.) Good. And Emma, since we are going to be working together, maybe it's a good idea if you come and stay with me. I could move my office here. What do you think? (she signs) Good idea? I think it is too. I know it is. (pause) Emma, show me how to say Merry Christmas. (She shows him and he signs.) Merry Christmas, Princess.

Emma: (signs) Merry Christmas, Big Daddy!

Emmett: Emma, now teach me how to say "I love you." (She pauses, then gives him a big hug. After a moment, finally he wraps his arms around her also.)

Emmett: Oh yes, of course. Thank you Emma, and—I love you too. (He squeezes her tighter.)

(They hug until the carolers finish singing "Silent Night," at which time they blow out their candles, and the stage lights fade simultaneously.)

THE END

GLOSSARY

Action: The dramatic events that occur due to the play's conflict or conflicts.

Arena Stage: Sometimes referred to as "theatre in the round," this stage has audience members on all sides of the actor.

Backstage: The areas off of or behind the performance space that are used for props, technical crews, and dressing rooms.

Barn Doors: Panels or "sides" that fasten to a spotlight that give better control over the shape and direction of the light.

Beat: The variation in a scene's mood, or the turn in a character's action—any scene can have dozens of beats, but each beat must have an objective (see objective).

Blackout: Stagelights are brought all the way down to total darkness in between scenes allowing performers to exit the stage unseen (see glowtape).

Blocking: The choreography of a play in which the actors and director work together to find the most comfortable places for standing, sitting, and other more specific stage movements that occur during natural dialogue.

Cast: The group of actresses and actors who perform your play.

Caterer: The one who coordinates and provides the dinner for your Dinner Theatre.

Center Stage: (CS) The middle of the performance area—since most of your play's traffic will pass through this spot, this is usually an ideal location for a hanging microphone and some general lighting.

Character: A person from your play's story (The actors learn their characters, and while onstage they stay "in character.").

Climax: All conflicts, great and small, lead to this turning point in your play when a character battles himself, or another character, in a confrontation that signifies the resolution of the play. (See conflict and resolution.)

Comedy: A play that is mainly humorous in its treatment of character and theme.

Conflict: Introduced very early in the storyline, this is the problem or obstacle that your audience will worry about throughout the play. The conflict may be between two characters, "man against man," or it can also be "man against nature," "man against himself," or "man against God." A play can have more than one conflict.

Costume Designer: One who shares creative control with the director over the design and production of a play's costume needs.

Crew: The technical and production personnel that work alongside the cast to enhance their performances through the use of lights, sound, costumes, makeup, etc. (See Chapter 7 for a complete list and definitions of individual technical and production crews necessary to produce a Dinner Theatre.)

Counter-cross: Coordinated stage movements between actors in which they may even temporarily cross in front of each other.

Cross: An actor's stage movement. ("Please *cross* centerstage to the table.")

Cue Line: The last line spoken before another actor speaks.

Curtain Call: Following the very end of the play, the final segment to the production in which the actors take the stage for their bows and applause.

Cyclorama: Also referred to as a *cyc*, this large surface at the back of a stage displays projected images or lights for special effect.

Dimmer Board: A lighting device used as a controlling tool in gradually raising and lowering the brightness of stagelights.

Dinner Theatre: A type of live entertainment in which audience members eat a catered meal and then watch a one or two-act play. Still confused? Read this book!

Downstage: (DS) The front of the performance area—from the actor's point of view, he must move downstage to get closer to the audience (See upstage.)

Drama: A type of play that explores situation conflict and emotion in a reflective fashion—although dramas can contain comedy, they tend to be more sober-sided.

Dress Rehearsal: A play's last few rehearsals that incorporate the actors, lights, sound, costumes, props, and every other area of technical production—the final dress rehearsal should be considered a performance to prepare the cast and crew mentally for their first live performance.

Ellipsoidal: A projector in which the exact direction of light can be easily pinpointed.

Evolution of Characters: The natural transformations that occur in a character from a play's beginning until its end.

Flats: Scenery located behind the actors that encloses the performance area. (Flats can be easily made by first nailing together a rectangular wooden frame that measures approximately 4' × 8'. Then using a staple gun, stretch white muslin material across the entire area. Finally, make a mixture of half glue and water and with the use of a roller, paint the entire flat surface. When it dries, you will have a very durable, canvas-like material to paint for your backdrop. These flats, if stored properly, can be reused from year to year, sometimes painted with a solid background color, and at other times displaying a tropical forest background.)

Follow-spot: A portable or mounted spotlight capable of following an actor's every move on stage when manually operated.

Fresnel: A spotlight named for the lens it holds.

Gels: Also called gel frames, these are colored frames attached to the front of a spotlight, projecting any desired color.

Glowtape: Glow-in-the-dark tape that lights a path for easy exits during blackouts.

Inherent Theme: The main idea behind your story or the internal message your audience will remember.

Intermission: A break or recess, usually ten minutes in length, in between the first and second acts of a play.

Lekos: A projector light with easy control of exact light direction.

Life-like Dialogue: Every play contains words. However, memorable plays have realistic dialogue that springs forth from realistic characters.

Melodrama: Although this art form originally meant the use of music with drama, it eventually became more well-known for its use of panic, despair, and relief in its sensational, suspenseful stories (i.e., we've all seen a play or movie with a damsel in distress tied to a railroad track. Just as the train approaches, to the sound of intense piano music, her dashing hero rescues her barely in time!)

Objective: A character's goal, although not necessarily just for the entire plot. For instance, each stage movement, each beat, must have an objective. If a character stands and crosses to the opposite side of the stage, he must have an objective to do so. Without a reason to cross, for example to pick up a ringing phone, his stage movement looks unnatural and premeditated.

Off-stage: Any area other than the main performance area.

One-act Play: Usually a 45-to-60 minute play with no intermission.

Pars: Round lights, about two feet in length with built-in reflectors in the bulb. They come in sizes of 48, 56, and 64.

Plot: It comprises the stepping stones of your play or how the action of your drama unfolds from beginning to end.

Props: "Properties," the hand-held objects that aid actors in portraying their characters. (i.e., a walking cane, a bouquet of flowers, a tray of food, etc.)

Prop table: A backstage table which displays all props and is managed by a properties manager. The prop manager assists the actors with their props upon their exits and entrances.

Proscenium Stage: This stage allows audience viewing from only one side of the stage, with the other three sides contained.

Rehearsal Schedule: Created by the director, this list includes rehearsal dates, rehearsal times, and what scenes will be rehearsed.

Resolution: The conclusion of the conflict. The way in which your narrative resolves itself.

Scrim: Used as a curtain and a backdrop, this thin piece of fabric remains an obscure barrier hiding the actors behind it when it is lit from the front. When these lights are lowered and some back lights are raised, the scrim becomes transparent, instantly revealing the action behind it.

Setting: The geographical place, central location, and time in which your storyline takes place.

Stage Left (SL): Stage directions are always given, keeping the actor's perspective in mind. When he is on-stage facing the audience, moving stage left indicates a move to his left.

Stage Right (SR): When an actor is onstage facing the audience, moving stage right indicates a move to his right.

Storyline: SETTING / TIMELESS CHARACTERS / OBSTACLE(S) / RESOLU-TION(S) / YAWLESS PLOT / LIFE-LIKE DIALOGUE / INHERENT THEME / NATURAL PROGRESSIONS / EVOLUTION OF CHARACTERS. (A formula discussed at length in Chapter 3, Get Ready . . . Set . . . Write!)

Story Question: This is the conflict that is introduced very early in the storyline, giving the audience or reader of the play something to "worry about" until the resolution occurs.

Subplot: A secondary or smaller conflict within the play that intensifies the main plot without distracting from it.

Subtext: Information revealed onstage about a character's previous actions offstage.

Tablework: The first steps in rehearsing a play. The cast is seated, and with scripts in hand, makes extensive notes regarding subtext, objectives, character, scene progressions, etc.

Thrust Stage: A stage including an area that protrudes or "thrusts' out into the audience.

Two-act Play: A play with an intermission dividing Act One and Act Two. Usually Act One is approximately 45-60 minutes in length, and the Second Act is a bit shorter. There is no rule to this, however.

Upstage (US): When an actor is downstage he is at the front of the stage closest to the audience. As he moves *upstage,* he makes his way to the back of the stage. Theatre history includes the theory that Elizabethan stages were built on a slant and that actors actually had to walk "upstage" and then back down the stage.

Wet-tech Rehearsal: When a play has been rehearsed and is "performable" the technical crews are allowed to attend this special rehearsal which gives them their first opportunity to set lights, sound, and other special effects.

DRAMATIC PUBLISHING COMPANIES

(CHECK THE MENTIONED CITY'S DIRECTORY ASSISTANCE FOR THE PUBLISHING COM-
PANY NEEDED SINCE PHONE NUMBERS AND ADDRESSES MAY CHANGE. A LIST OF
HOW TO BEST UTILIZE THESE COMPANIES IS EXPLAINED IN CHAPTER 2.)

Baker's Plays of Boston, Massachusetts
Broadman & Holman Publishers of Nashville, Tennessee
The Coach House Press, Inc., of Chicago, Illinois
Contemporary Drama Service of Downers Grove, Illinois
Convention Press of Nashville, Tennessee
Drama Book Shoppe of New York, New York
The Dramatic Book Publishers of New York, New York
The Dramatic Publishing Company of Chicago, Illinois
Dramatists Play Service, Inc. of New York, New York
Performance Publishing of Elgin, Illinois
Pioneer Drama Service of Denver, Colorado
Samuel French, Inc. of New York, New York
Stage Magic Plays of Schulenburg, Texas
Word Ministry Resources of Dallas, Texas